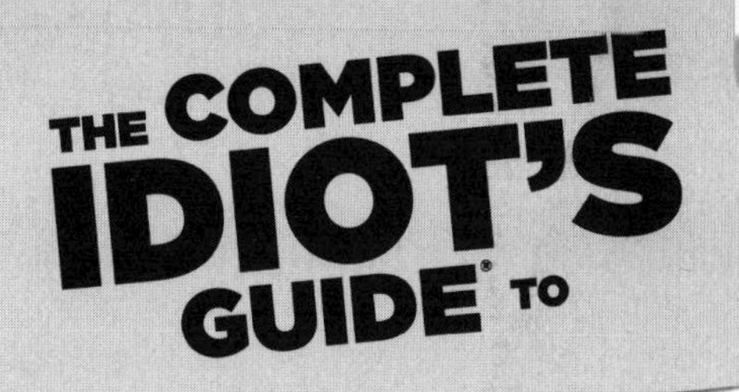

The Acid Reflux Diet

by Maria A. Bella, MS, RD, CDN

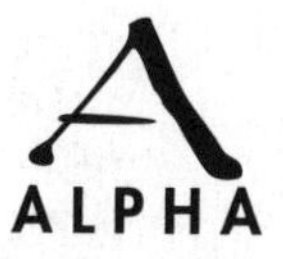

A member of Penguin Group (USA) Inc.

ALPHA BOOKS

Published by the Penguin Group

Penguin Group (USA) Inc., 375 Hudson Street, New York, New York 10014, USA

Penguin Group (Canada), 90 Eglinton Avenue East, Suite 700, Toronto, Ontario M4P 2Y3, Canada (a division of Pearson Penguin Canada Inc.)

Penguin Books Ltd., 80 Strand, London WC2R 0RL, England

Penguin Ireland, 25 St. Stephen's Green, Dublin 2, Ireland (a division of Penguin Books Ltd.)

Penguin Group (Australia), 250 Camberwell Road, Camberwell, Victoria 3124, Australia (a division of Pearson Australia Group Pty. Ltd.)

Penguin Books India Pvt. Ltd., 11 Community Centre, Panchsheel Park, New Delhi—110 017, India

Penguin Group (NZ), 67 Apollo Drive, Rosedale, North Shore, Auckland 1311, New Zealand (a division of Pearson New Zealand Ltd.)

Penguin Books (South Africa) (Pty.) Ltd., 24 Sturdee Avenue, Rosebank, Johannesburg 2196, South Africa

Penguin Books Ltd., Registered Offices: 80 Strand, London WC2R 0RL, England

International Standard Book Number: 978-1-61564-140-6
Library of Congress Catalog Card Number: 2011910192

14 13 12 8 7 6 5 4 3 2 1

Interpretation of the printing code: The rightmost number of the first series of numbers is the year of the book's printing; the rightmost number of the second series of numbers is the number of the book's printing. For example, a printing code of 12-1 shows that the first printing occurred in 2012.

Printed in the United States of America

Publisher: *Marie Butler-Knight*
Associate Publisher: *Mike Sanders*
Executive Managing Editor: *Billy Fields*
Senior Development Editor: *Christy Wagner*
Senior Acquisitions Editors: *Brook Farling, Paul Dinas*
Senior Production Editor: *Kayla Dugger*
Copy Editor: *Amy Lepore*
Cover Designer: *Kurt Owens*
Book Designers: *William Thomas, Rebecca Batchelor*
Indexer: *Julie Bess*
Layout: *Ayanna Lacey*
Senior Proofreader: *Laura Caddell*

This book is dedicated to my wise parents, my beautiful sister, and my loving husband.

Contents

Appendixes

Introduction

Is this your first time experiencing acid reflux symptoms, or are you a lifelong sufferer? Whichever category you fall into, you've come to the right place. This book is based on the latest cutting-edge, scientific information combined with practical advice to help you live easier with acid reflux—and you can start implementing it into your life today!

Many dietary and physiological factors can contribute to the development of acid reflux. This comprehensive guide shows you which factors put you at risk and what changes can alleviate your symptoms. It empowers you with the tools and information to handle any party preparation, social occasion, and travel situation—all 100 percent free of acid reflux symptoms.

How to Use This Book

I've divided this book into four parts. I suggest reading all the parts once and then using certain parts such as tables, travel tips, and recipes as a reference you can keep coming back to. Here's what you'll find:

Part 1, A Closer Look at Acid Reflux, gives you a detailed introduction to the gastrointestinal tract and acid reflux. Between old wives' tales and a plethora of online information, it's often hard to decipher facts from fiction. Part 1 arms you with a thorough understanding of what causes acid reflux and how you can say good-bye to it.

Part 2, Ensuring Your Success on the Acid Reflux Diet, shows you how fun and sustainable following an acid reflux diet can be. Every person is different, and a one-size approach does not fit all. In Part 2, I help you identify your triggers and educate you on creating a well-balanced diet to keep acid reflux at bay. I also share tips for making sense of exercise and sports nutrition and how it relates to acid reflux.

Part 3, Cooking and Dining Out Strategies, helps you handle eating in any social situation, navigate restaurant menus with ease, and enjoy dining out while on vacation, all reflux free.

In **Part 4, Recipes for Reflux-Free Living,** I provide over 140 delicious recipes, from breakfast to dessert, that have been specifically created with acid reflux–friendly ingredients. Whether you're an expert cook or only use your stove for reheating leftovers, there's a recipe in Part 4 for you! You can use these recipes as is, or customize them for a personalized menu.

Extras

In every chapter, you'll notice fun and useful sidebars. Here's what to look for:

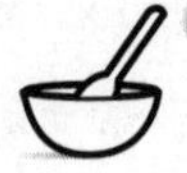

DEFINITION

These sidebars provide definitions of some important scientific terms and cooking terminology.

ACID ALERT

Check out these warnings for extra information about possible acid reflux triggers. Keeping track of these alerts may uncover hidden reflux triggers you've not thought of before.

TUMMY TAMER

Turn to these sidebars for tips on how to make things easier, healthier, and tastier.

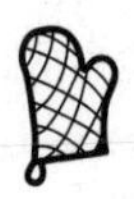

COOLER TALK

Check out these sidebars filled with fun facts and useful information.

Acknowledgments

Many special thanks to all who have made this book possible. First, I am forever indebted to my wonderful agent, Jessica Faust, and two of the most brilliant editorial experts, Brook Farling and Christy Wagner, for making this project possible. Your kindness and ongoing feedback are appreciated more than you know.

Sincere thanks to Colin J. Powers, MD, FACS, FASMBS, at the Center for Bariatric Surgical Specialties at North Shore LIJ Healthcare System for his unconditional support, his belief in my ability to reach my dreams, and for always being there to help. Thanks to Tara Miller, MS, RD, CDN—an amazing dietitian—for being such a great mentor. Special thanks to Dr. James Underberg at the Murray Hill Practice Group for all his referrals and entrusting me with his patients.

Many thanks to two of the smartest dietitians and nutrition experts, Simone Harounian, MS, RD, CDN, and Elaine Tang, RD, for all the hard work and wisdom contributed to this project. I also thank my graduate student interns—Melissa Arana, Amanda Chatham, Jennifer Cheon, Maegan McCully, and Khadiga Spahi. Your research has been invaluable to me in writing this book.

Above and beyond, a huge thank you goes out to my parents—you have given me the strength to reach for the stars! Thanks to my grandmother for always inspiring me with words of wisdom and to my grandfather, a lifelong acid reflux sufferer, for spending hours on the phone helping me develop delicious recipes. A special thanks to my husband for his understanding, help, and tremendous patience!

Trademarks

Part 1

A Closer Look at Acid Reflux

When you realize how your body works, you can better understand what causes acid reflux and how it affects you. In Part 1, I help you recognize your symptoms, know when to seek professional help, and select your best course of treatment. When you have the foundation to understand your acid reflux symptoms, you can learn how to alleviate them by following a specific diet.

Weight management with acid reflux can present a unique challenge. Many diet foods are loaded with reflux triggers, and stomach discomfort may make it difficult to determine when you're truly hungry. To round out Part 1, I give you a chapter on weight management that explains the connection between weight and reflux and gives you the tools to develop your own best diet tailored to your personal goals.

What Causes Acid Reflux?

Chapter

1

In This Chapter

- Symptoms of acid reflux
- How and why of acid reflux
- Diagnosing acid reflux
- What acid reflux is not—close siblings

Approximately 10 million adults in the United States suffer from acid reflux, a painful condition of stomach acid backing up into the esophagus. When it comes to dealing with acid reflux, understanding the physiology of your gastrointestinal tract is just as important as following a diet to keep acid reflux at bay. This knowledge can also help you select the best treatment options for your condition.

In this chapter, you learn what acid reflux really is and how it really feels. Understanding the physiology behind acid reflux helps you see why it happens in your body and how to differentiate acid reflux from similar conditions. Finally, this chapter explains what tests doctors perform to diagnose this condition.

Symptoms of Acid Reflux

The main symptom of acid reflux is heartburn. This burning sensation occurs in the lower part of the middle of the chest, behind the breastbone, and can extend to the middle of the abdomen. The pain can rise from the stomach and radiate to the neck, the throat, and sometimes even the back. Heartburn mostly occurs after a meal, especially a large meal or one that consists of spicy, citrus-y, or fatty foods or is accompanied by chocolate or alcohol.

Regurgitation, or the feeling of sour or bitter-tasting acid backing up into the throat, may occur, too. You may feel unpleasant sensations such as indigestion, stomach discomfort, nausea after eating, bloating, or burping. You may also have acid reflux if you experience difficulty in swallowing, increased salivation, belching, severe pain that can radiate to the neck or jaw, and water brash (salty fluid in the mouth secreted from the salivary gland in response to acid reflux).

Finally, food getting stuck in your throat, painful swallowing, a sore throat, worsening dental disease, recurrent pneumonia, chronic sinusitis, waking up with choking sensation, persistent laryngitis, or hoarseness may also be a sign of acid reflux.

Now that you know what to look for, let's see how all this comes about, and what you can do to stop it from happening again.

The Basics of Digestion

It helps to understand how your body processes what you eat and exactly where and how acid reflux occurs in the digestion process. Digestion begins as soon as you put a piece of food in your mouth. Your teeth grind and crush the food into smaller and smaller pieces until only particles remain. The smaller the bits, the easier the stomach can process them. As your teeth break down the food, the saliva released from your salivary glands, from under your tongue and the sides of your mouth, moistens and lubricates the food particles into a food mass.

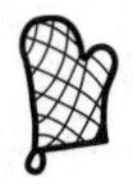

COOLER TALK

Saliva contains many different enzymes, the most abundant of which is amylase. Amylase works in your mouth to break down starches into smaller molecules of sugar as they pass into your stomach. Once the amylase hits the acid in the stomach, it becomes inactive, allowing other digestion processes to take over.

Your tongue helps move the food mass along to the back of your mouth, where it then makes its way to the pharynx to begin the swallowing phase. Up until the food mass reaches the back of your mouth, digestion is still voluntary. You have total control of swallowing and moving your tongue and pushing the food mass to the back of your throat. Once the food mass is pushed back, you lose control of digestion and the involuntary process begins.

A wavelike movement called peristalsis pushes the food more rapidly down the esophagus, the tube that connects your mouth to your stomach. Before the food mass enters the stomach, it bypasses the lower esophageal sphincter (LES), which acts like a swinging one-way door, allowing food to enter the stomach but preventing it from coming back into the esophagus. This barrier helps prevent the reflux of food and liquids from the stomach into the esophagus.

In the Stomach

Speaking of the stomach, that's where the food goes next. The stomach has a few major functions, one of which is temporary storage. After a big meal, the stomach can hold food for a while. During that time, the food is pushed forward with wavelike contractions. The movement mixes the food with different types of stomach liquids, digestive enzymes, and different types of secretions. One type of secretion is hydrochloric acid (HCl). Others include enzymes like protease, which breaks down protein, and lipase, which breaks down fat.

During all this, the stomach also liquefies the contents of the food into *chyme* so it's ready for the small intestine.

DEFINITION

Chyme is a semifluid consisting of partially digested food, gastric juices, and digestive enzymes. Chyme passes from the stomach into the small intestine for further digestion.

The stomach digests nutrients such as protein from your food. HCl is an important ingredient for digestion because it activates the pepsin, which is secreted by the cells that line the stomach, to help digest protein. HCl also helps destroy all the different types of microorganisms eaten with the food. The acid is so strong—it has pH of 1 through 4—it greatly decreases the amount of microorganisms like bacteria and molds that may cause illness.

At the end of the stomach, there's another sphincter called the pyloric sphincter that helps control the emptying of the stomach contents into the small intestine. The pyloric sphincter helps prevent the backflow of stuff from the small intestine into the stomach, just like the LES does between the stomach and the esophagus. Emotional changes, certain food choices, and the activity in the digestive system can all affect the function of the sphincters.

A solid meal may take about 2 or 3 hours after it's been eaten to pass through your stomach and empty into the small intestine. A liquid meal empties much faster, at about 1 or 2 hours. Food in the small intestine and different types of hormones that regulate digestion may also change the rate at which the stomach empties.

Certain types of food items and beverages can modify the LES's pressure system, and can allow reflux of the stomach contents into the esophagus. Stomach secretions are extremely acidic and, therefore, damage the outside mucosal layers of esophagus when they're regurgitated back from the stomach. Also, *hyperosmolaric* foods, such as sugary drinks, may exacerbate these effects.

DEFINITION

Hyperosmolarity refers to the increased concentration of the solute, for instance high concentrations of sugar in the blood. Hyperosmolaric foods include those high in sugar or fat.

In the Small Intestine and Beyond

Most of the digestion of food and nutrients happens in the small intestine. It's about 20 feet long and is divided into three sections: the duodenum, the jejunum, and the ileum. Most of the breakdown and absorption of food takes place in the duodenum and the beginning of the jejunum.

When the chyme first hits the duodenum, it's still acidic from the stomach's HCl. The chyme mixes with all the juices released in the duodenum and the pancreas. The pancreas, an organ connected to the small intestine by a small tube, secretes fluid and enzymes that digest all the major nutrients. The fluid, called bicarbonate, has the opposite effect of HCl and begins to neutralize the acidic chyme. Once it's neutralized, the enzymes of the small intestine work better.

The partially digested food stimulates hormones that then stimulate the secretion of enzymes and fluids. This chain reaction tells your body you're full and then starts moving the food along the intestine. The liver and gallbladder are also connected to the small intestine and release bile that emulsifies and helps break down and absorb fat.

The jejunum is lined with cells that absorb carbohydrates and proteins. The amino acids from protein, sugar from carbohydrates, fatty acids, and some vitamins and minerals are absorbed and brought into the bloodstream where the nutrients travel all over the body for fuel.

At the end of the small intestine, you can find the ileum. Here fat and bile salts are absorbed, as well as vitamins like A, D, K, E, and B_{12}. After they're absorbed, they're immediately taken into the bloodstream to distribute to the rest of the body. It takes about 3 to 8 hours to move contents along the small intestine.

The ileocecal valve connects the ileum with the large intestine. This valve, like the two sphincters discussed earlier, prevents the backflow of the liquids into the small intestine. The large intestine carries the nondigestible contents to the colon for excretion.

Who's at Risk for Acid Reflux?

Certain ages and groups are more prone to reflux than others. Pregnant women, infants and children, and the elderly are the top three at-risk categories. Let's take a look at why.

Pregnant Women

Two out of three women experience acid reflux during their pregnancy. This may be due to several factors. During pregnancy, the placenta produces a hormone called progesterone. Progesterone relaxes the LES, and that can allow stomach acid to backflow into the esophagus. Progesterone also can slow down peristalsis (the involuntary muscle contraction of the esophagus), making it difficult to continue the process of digestion. It takes much longer.

The growing and enlarged uterus crowds the stomach and can push the stomach acid upward toward the esophagus, especially with the LES more relaxed. Women who experience acid reflux before pregnancy are more prone to experience more severe symptoms while they're pregnant. Symptoms may improve once the baby is born.

Complications from acid reflux are rare, however, and when they occur, it's mostly inflammation of the esophagus.

Infants and Children

Most infants experience gastroesophageal reflux in some form; however, it's often overlooked because infants cannot articulate their symptoms. Most infants may experience gastroesophageal reflux (GER) and are healthy even if they vomit or spit up frequently. Infants usually outgrow this by their first birthday.

If it continues past the first year, it may be diagnosed as GERD. Symptoms include regurgitation, nausea, heartburn, coughing, laryngitis, respiratory problems like wheezing, asthma, pneumonia, or blood in stool.

To determine if your child has reflux, watch her expression or posture. She might be irritable during or after a feeding, or she might even arch her back. In extreme cases of acid reflux, the child may refuse to eat.

Treatment plans include burping the infant several times during the feeding and keeping her in an upright position for 30 minutes after a feeding. Your physician may prescribe medication if the symptoms persist.

The Elderly

Two in three adults over age 65 experience acid reflux. This population may have lower-functioning esophageal muscles or a decrease in the amount of saliva made in their mouth, which helps neutralize the acid. The elderly are often on more medication, and some side effects of certain medications may make the LES not as strong.

Older adults may experience a more severe form of acid reflux even though the symptoms are less bothersome. Their symptoms may not be as severe possibly due to decrease in pain perception at that stage of life.

Certain diseases such as erosive esophagitis, peptic stricture, Barrett's esophagitis, pulmonary complications, and iron deficiency anemia may also complicate how badly reflux may occur or its associated symptoms.

Getting Help

If you experience long-term acid reflux and don't treat it, it can cause even more serious complications. Acid from the stomach can damage whatever tissue it hits. Overexposure to acid can lead to bleeding or ulcers. Once the bleeding scars, strictures can develop that narrow your esophagus, making it more difficult to swallow. Barrett's esophagus is a condition of long-term acid reflux complication where the cells in the esophagus lining become disfigured and discolored. Over time, these cells may become cancerous. Without a doubt, it's very important to contact your physician for proper handling of your symptoms before they get worse.

Your primary care physician may be a great place to start. Describe your symptoms thoroughly, and ask for a referral to an appropriate specialist if necessary. Also, a registered dietitian can be your best ally in developing a meal plan tailored to your diagnosis and your goals.

TUMMY TAMER

Alert your dietitian about the name of your physician and vice versa for continuity of care. Two brains are better than one, and this will ensure that everybody is on the same page when it comes to your treatment.

Diagnosing Acid Reflux

Acid reflux becomes gastroesophageal reflux disorder (GERD) when the symptoms are bothersome or cause injury to the esophagus. At this point, the esophagus cannot clear away the acid as quickly to prevent longer contact with the acidic refluxed contents. The total amount of reflux required to diagnose GERD differs with each person. As a rule of thumb, when heartburn occurs at least two or three times a week, it is called GERD.

GERD is a condition in which irritation and inflammation of the esophagus can lead to reflux of gastric acid into the esophagus. GERD happens when the gastric contents, which mostly consist of HCl and pepsin, are refluxed into the esophagus frequently or in extreme quantity. It can also occur when the refluxed gastric contents do not cause esophageal contractions to push the contents back to the stomach.

Heartburn occurs when gastric acid is in contact with the lining of the esophagus in large quantities and for a long time. There are mild and severe cases of GERD. Mild cases include the feeling of heartburn but with a normal lining of the esophagus (esophageal mucosa). More severe forms of GERD include an inflamed and ulcerated lining of the esophagus, vomiting, and difficulty swallowing.

Many times tests aren't necessary to diagnose GERD because frequent heartburn and acid regurgitation are enough to figure out what's happening. However, it's imperative that your primary care physician perform a physical examination and ask questions about your health. You should provide him or her with your information, especially about your symptoms. Your doctor may treat the symptoms with a prescription medication intended to reduce or block acid production. If these symptoms are not improved with lifestyle changes or the prescription medication, additional tests may be needed to determine what's going on.

Let's take a look at a few of these tests:

The simplest method is the *proton pump inhibitor (PPI) test*, in which medication is given to suppress production of acid in the stomach and resulting symptoms are closely monitored. This is the most common first diagnostic test given when the patient is experiencing classic reflux symptoms. If the symptoms disappear with the medication but then return once the medication is no longer administered, GERD is diagnosed.

The *barium swallow radiograph* is an x-ray used to spot any abnormalities with swallowing and the movement of the food down the esophagus and into the stomach. If your doctor orders a barium swallow radiograph, you'll drink a barium solution and x-rays will be taken. This test identifies strictures, narrowing of the esophagus, or even the presence of ulcers. Mild irritation due to acid reflux is not shown, so it's not a good indicator for infrequent bouts of acid reflux.

The *upper endoscopy exam* is more accurate than the barium swallow. Your throat is numbed, and you're sedated to be more at ease and calm. The physician slides the endoscope—a thin and flexible plastic tube with a light and a camera lens at the end—through your esophagus and into your stomach. The tiny camera shows the surface of your esophagus so your doctor can search for any abnormalities through a video monitor.

Esophageal pH monitoring is a procedure in which a small tube is inserted into your esophagus for 24 to 48 hours. While you go about your normal daily activities, this tube measures when and how much acid is refluxed into your esophagus. This procedure is particularly helpful to use along with a *food diary*. It helps connect the acid reflux episodes with the triggers. This is the most sensitive test for GERD.

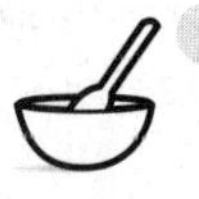

DEFINITION

A **food diary** is a record of what foods were eaten, how much, and at what time.

Esophageal manometry is the assessment of how well your LES contracts and relaxes, and how well food moves down into your stomach. With this procedure, you swallow a tube that measures the muscle contractions of your esophagus. This procedure determines if your LES is functioning properly. Generally, this test is not indicated in the evaluation of uncomplicated GERD. However, this test is recommended for people with unclear diagnosis of GERD or any complication of the esophagus.

What Acid Reflux Is Not

Many times acid reflux symptoms are confused with other conditions that may need immediate care. Let's take a look at some conditions that may be related to or have similar symptoms as acid reflux, but are not.

Gastritis is the inflammation, irritation, or swelling of the lining of the stomach. The cells that make up this lining are extremely important for digestion. They produce acid and enzymes that help break down the food for digestion. The mucus in the stomach helps protect the stomach lining from the acid. When the lining is inflamed, it produces less acid, enzymes, and mucus.

Inflammation is often the result of an infection with the same bacterium associated with most stomach ulcers, H. pylori. The pain is usually in the upper abdomen, much like acid reflux. Most people with gastritis do not experience any symptoms.

Irritable bowel syndrome (IBS) is a disorder characterized by abdominal pain, cramps, bloating, diarrhea, and constipation. This condition does not permanently harm the intestines, but it does cause many uncomfortable symptoms for people with this diagnosis. Symptoms are mostly controlled with diet, stress management, and prescription medication. The peristaltic movement that occurs throughout the digestive tract may not be as active in the area of the colon. The colon also may not respond well to certain foods or stress.

Esophageal dysmotility is a condition characterized by a decrease in the contraction and movement of muscles in the esophagus. Many different factors can be contributing causes, but age, the prolonged effect of acid reflux, diabetes, scleroderma, Parkinson's disease, ALS, thyroid disease, and certain drugs are the main culprits. Symptoms can be similar to GERD and include heartburn, dysphagia, regurgitation, and coughing. It's particularly important to diagnose esophageal dysmotility because the common symptoms do not improve with traditional GERD medication like PPIs, antacids, or lifestyle changes.

Ulcers, or peptic ulcers, are open sores that develop inside the lining of the esophagus, stomach, or upper portion of the small intestine. The most common symptom is abdominal pain, but others may include burning in the middle upper stomach between meals or at night, bloating, heartburn, nausea, or vomiting. Ulcers form for many reasons. An ulcer can be the end result of an imbalance between digestive fluids in the stomach and the duodenum. Ulcers also can be due to infection because of the bacterium H. pylori and can be caused by painkillers like nonsteroidal anti-inflammatory drugs (NSAIDs) including aspirin, naproxen, and ibuprofen.

The Least You Need to Know

- Recognizing the symptoms of acid reflux—heartburn, burping, lower chest pain after a meal, difficulty in swallowing, increased salivation, belching, severe pain that can radiate to the neck or jaw—helps you know when to seek professional help.
- Slow movement of food through the digestive tract increases chances of acid reflux. Spicy, acidic, and fatty foods all contribute to the condition.
- Even though some symptoms may be similar, acid reflux is different from IBS, gastritis, ulcers, and esophageal dysmotility.
- Certain demographics are more susceptible to acid reflux than others, especially infants and children, pregnant women, and the elderly.

Chapter 2

Treating and Relieving Acid Reflux

In This Chapter

- Change your diet, improve acid reflux symptoms
- The effect of sleep, stress, smoking, and exercise on acid reflux
- Herbal and medical remedies for acid reflux
- Surgical intervention in treatment of acid reflux

Now that you know what causes acid reflux, let's look at how you can find relief from it. In this chapter, I discuss treatments commonly used for quelling the painful symptoms of acid reflux.

The first line of therapy is generally lifestyle adjustments. Monitoring your diet, stopping smoking, managing stress, and wearing looser clothing often help. Some home remedies might also give you some relief. But if making diet and other adjustments doesn't significantly improve your symptoms, it's time to speak with your health-care provider. He or she may prescribe medication or recommend other procedures such as surgery (in rare cases) that can provide relief.

Pain-Relieving Lifestyle Adjustments

Lifestyle modification is the first and foremost step to help you take control of your battle with acid reflux. Simple lifestyle adjustments can significantly help relieve acid reflux symptoms. These changes focus on improving the function of the esophagus—making sure the acid is cleared into the stomach, minimizing the incidence of reflux events, cessation of smoking, and avoiding late meals.

If you have a mild case of acid reflux, changes to your diet could be an easy solution to your problem. Changing to healthy foods, especially whole foods or those as close to nature as possible, is a simple first step. Foods that come packaged or don't have an expiration date are generally very processed and loaded with chemicals and artificial ingredients. Those types of foods exacerbate acid reflux because they interfere with proper digestion and movement of food through the digestive tract. Opt for a balanced diet of healthy foods from all food groups, such as whole grains, fruits, vegetables, low- or nonfat dairy, lean meats and poultry, and limited quantities of healthy sources of fats like vegetable oil, nuts, and seeds.

In addition to *what* you eat, *when* you eat makes a difference. Space out your meals through the day, eating smaller and more frequent meals. Take the time to eat slowly, too—after all, eating should be an enjoyable process! Chew your food thoroughly so your stomach doesn't have to work as hard to digest it and, therefore, doesn't have to produce as much acid. Be sure not to eat in the 2 or 3 hours before you lay down. It's better if you give food enough time to digest and empty your stomach contents.

TUMMY TAMER

It can be helpful to keep a heartburn diary to remember what foods you eat and at what times to see what triggers your reflux. Once you learn what foods and beverages exacerbate your symptoms, you can avoid them. This also helps keep you accountable for the number of calories and the quality of the food you eat.

Furthermore, exercise will help with weight loss. Alone, being overweight dramatically increases the chances of developing acid reflux. If your weight is under control, it can help strengthen your muscles. (Turn to Chapter 7 for more on exercise.)

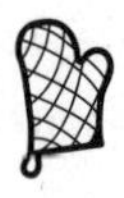

COOLER TALK

A body mass index (BMI) greater than 25 (overweight and obese category) makes it 2.5 to 3 times more likely that you'll develop GERD.

Now let's take a look at what I call the "magic four": smoking, stress, sleep, and style. You might not think smoking, stress management, what you do before and during sleep, and the type of clothing you wear around your waist would make a difference to your acid reflux, but they do.

Quitting Smoking

Smoking cigarettes can affect your acid reflux in more ways than one. For starters, smoking decreases salivation, and saliva, if you remember from Chapter 1, is important in helping neutralize refluxed acid. Smoking also lowers the pressure in the lower esophageal sphincter (LES) and can aggravate coughing that causes more episodes of acid reflux in the esophagus. Quitting smoking can significantly reduce or eliminate your acid reflux symptoms.

Many methods are available to help you quit smoking. Speak with your doctor; he or she can point you in the right direction and help you with options such as support groups, hypnosis, acupuncture, or medication for quitting. Over-the-counter (OTC) smoking-cessation aids such as gum, lozenges, patches, and nasal sprays are available in drug stores and may help you quit.

Managing Stress

Although there's no proven link between stress and acid reflux, stress can be related to increased incidence of acid reflux. Under stressful conditions, for example, people are more likely to eat more, especially comfort food, which is more likely to be higher in fat. Stress also may cause people to drink alcohol, smoke, or sleep less. All these are triggers of acid reflux.

Plus, under stressful conditions, blood flow goes more toward the muscles in the arms and the legs, meaning less blood is available for the stomach. Therefore, food is digested more slowly and gastric emptying decreases, making food lingering in the stomach more apt to be refluxed.

Stressful conditions also trigger the "fight or flight" response. During these times, there's an immediate decrease in the energy and oxygen used by the digestive tract, which slows down digestion, leaving food in the stomach for a longer period of time.

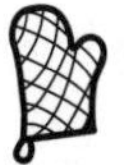

COOLER TALK

Stress is derived from the Greek word *stringere,* which translates to "pull tight."

Regardless of whether stress has an impact on acid reflux or not, stress reduction is a healthy approach to your overall well-being. Using relaxation techniques is beneficial no matter what your ailment. Studies have shown that patients who use relaxation techniques have significantly lower heart rates, less anxiety, significantly decrease reflux symptoms, and lower esophageal acid exposure than patients who do not practice relaxation techniques.

Exercise also relieves stress while helping with weight loss. Massage therapy, deep breathing, visualization, yoga, and meditation are also fantastic sources of stress relief.

Anyone can meditate. It's as simple as taking 5 minutes to relax and shut off your mind to outside disturbances. Use this time to treat yourself to serenity, and take your mind out of any stresses of the day. It only takes 5 minutes! Here's how:

1. Find a quiet, comfortable area, such as a private spot in the office, at a park, or even at home. Get into a comfortable position, and sit with your spine straight, cross-legged if you can, on a chair or even on the grass.
2. Find something to focus on. Pick a meaningful word or phrase, and repeat it. Or even focus on an object like a flower or a doorknob. Or you can close your eyes.
3. While you're sitting in comfort and relaxation, thoughts may come to you as distractions, but don't worry about them. Accept them, and return to what you've been focusing on.

Don't get frustrated if this isn't relaxing at first. It takes lots of practice, but the rewards are endless.

TUMMY TAMER

If you can't sit still for 5 minutes or more, consider practicing Tai Chi, or moving meditation. Tai Chi is an ancient martial art that combines slow movements and breathing techniques to cultivate and direct life energy, or chi.

Some Notes on Sleep

When you're in an upright position, the combination of swallowing your saliva and the force of gravity helps push acid reflux back into your stomach. When you're lying flat, however, especially when you're sleeping, you swallow less saliva and less gravity is at work. Plus, your LES might not be as strong as it is while you're awake. Because your body takes longer to push the acid down the GI tract while you sleep, acid is more likely to back up high in your esophagus or even in the back of your mouth. And deep sleep makes heartburn less obvious.

Most people experience heartburn 2 or 3 hours after meals, and some people wake up at night with heartburn. Studies show that people who have acid reflux have difficulty sleeping through the night and wake up often. Making changes in your eating and sleeping habits can help improve the symptoms you experience both right before you go to bed and during the night.

For example, you can raise your head and shoulders higher than your stomach so gravity can help keep down acid reflux. One way to do this is by elevating the head of your bed using 6- to 8-inch blocks under the legs. Or you might use a Styrofoam wedge under the head of your mattress. The wedge pillow supports and elevates your upper body, while gravity helps keep the acid down and makes breathing easier. Sleeping this way prevents the acid from burning your throat or esophagus and does not put any added pressure on your stomach.

ACID ALERT

Sleeping propped up with additional pillows under your head and shoulders causes an unnatural bend in the body, may increase pressure on your stomach, and ultimately worsens acid reflux.

Try to sleep on the left side of your body. Some studies have shown that this position is preferred over sleeping on the right side because of the way our bodies are designed. Your esophagus slightly curves, so sleeping on your left side makes the angle sharper, limiting the flow of stomach acid into the esophagus. When you sleep, try wearing loose clothing so you don't create any extra pressure on your stomach.

Before bedtime, establish a reflux-friendly routine. Avoid eating right before bedtime—keep a minimum of 2 or 3 hours between your meal time and bedtime, always sit straight when you're eating, and don't lie down or bend down immediately after a meal. Lying down on a full stomach can increase your chances of acid reflux. Be sure you maintain a regular and relaxing routine before bedtime. You can take a bath or shower, read a book, or even listen to some soothing music. Or take those 5 minutes and meditate!

Getting Dressed

The type of clothing you wear can affect your acid reflux, especially if you're overweight. Tight clothing can increase pressure in your abdominal area, which can force the contents of your stomach back up into your esophagus. You should be comfortable in whatever you wear. Be sure your garments are loose fitting. Tight belts, tight pants, and hosiery are fashion culprits of acid reflux.

TUMMY TAMER

If your infant or child experiences acid reflux, be sure none of her clothing is putting additional pressure on her abdominal area. One-piece clothing tends to be a great option.

Soothing Herbal and Plant-Derived Remedies

Herbal remedies can be effective in reducing acid reflux symptoms, but what might work for others might not work for you. Even though the jury is still out on the effectiveness of some herbal remedies, it's worth educating yourself. This noninvasive method of treatment may be the solution.

Licorice in the form of *deglycyrrhizinated licorice (DGL)* coats the stomach and esophagus by forming a soothing film, providing an extra layer of protection from the acid. It's thought to decrease inflammation and ulceration by decreasing the activity of pepsin in the body.

Aloe vera juice is often used to relieve heartburn. Try drinking $\frac{1}{4}$ cup aloe vera juice about 30 minutes before you eat. Although no studies confirm the effectiveness of aloe, it has been noted to soothe an irritated esophagus.

Slippery elm is an herb found in the inner bark of the tree. The gummy mucilage has been thought to coat the esophagus and decrease any inflammation.

Marshmallow is an old-fashioned remedy that also contains mucilage, helping soothe the lining of the esophagus. It also helps lower the acid level in the stomach. Herbalists recommend marshmallow in the form of its root tea.

Rice bran oil has been known to relieve acid reflux symptoms, but the evidence is limited.

Chewing *gum* between meals activates saliva, which is alkaline and stimulates peristalsis.

Bananas are also alkaline and are high in potassium. The soft texture and consistency soothes the irritated esophagus.

Meadowsweet helps the lining of the digestive tract. It is found to be a natural antacid and helps balance the ratio of stomach acid to digestive secretions.

German chamomile is a soothing herb that, once in the body, becomes a tonic to help support digestion.

Herbs can have serious side effects, and may interfere with some prescription medications, so ask your doctor about safe dosage before beginning any herbal remedy—for acid reflux or for any other ailment. Once you're cleared, you can find these remedies at your local supermarket or a health food store.

Prescription Medications

Your doctor might prescribe medication if you have moderate to severe symptoms of acid reflux, complications of GERD, or mild symptoms that don't respond to lifestyle modification. The key to taking prescription medication is to take the lowest dose possible for the shortest time possible while controlling symptoms and preventing complications. This helps limit the possible side effects of medications.

ACID ALERT

Whenever you're prescribed medication, it's important to let your medical provider know about any other medications, herbs, or supplements you may be taking so you can avoid drug-to-drug or drug-to-nutrient interaction. This may have life-threatening consequences if it goes unnoticed.

Medications That Can Help

OTC antacids are the first line of medication recommended for mild heartburn or mild symptoms of acid reflux because they work quickly to neutralize acid in the stomach and ease pain. Antacids are the combination of three salts—magnesium, calcium, and aluminum—plus a buffering agent like hydroxide or bicarbonate ion. Antacids you might find in the drugstore include Alka-Seltzer, Maalox (aluminum hydroxide, magnesium dyroxide), Mylanta (simethicone), Rolaids (calcium carbonate), Riopan (magaldrate), and Tums (calcium carbonate).

Side effects are generally minimal but may include diarrhea from magnesium salts or constipation from aluminum salts. Some antacids combine magnesium and aluminum to balance out the diarrhea and constipation.

Another OTC class of drugs is foaming agents that, as the name implies, coat and cover the stomach contents with foam, which prevents reflux. They work similarly to antacids, based on a mixture of neutralizers and buffering agents plus a gelling agent, to create a barrier that helps prevent the contents of the stomach from refluxing. Gaviscon is one example.

H2 blockers, also called H2-receptor antagonists, can be found both OTC and prescription strength. This medicine works to reduce the amount of acid the stomach produces by blocking histamine2, a chemical floating in the stomach that signals it to make acid. They don't relieve reflux as quickly as antacids, but they do provide short-term relief and are effective for about half of people with GERD. H2 blockers include drugs like Zantac (ranitidine), Pepcid (famotidine), Tagamet (cimetidine), and Axid (nizatidine).

Proton pump inhibitors (PPIs), prescription medications generally more effective than H2 blockers, are currently the best treatment option. They act by irreversibly blocking the proton pump of the parietal cells on the lining of the stomach. The proton pump is the last stage right before acid, or H+, is pumped out of the cells. Because this drug targets the last step in acid secretion and is irreversible, PPIs are thought to be more effective than H2 antagonists. They also relieve symptoms and heal the esophageal lining in almost all cases of GERD. PPIs include Prilosec (omeprazole), Zegerid (omeprazole and sodium bicarbonate), Prevacid (lansoprazole), Protonix (pantoprazole), Aciphex (rabeprazole), and Nexium (esomeprazole).

Your doctor will determine the type of PPI for you and the optimal dose. He or she will likely place you on a test run for about 8 weeks. Depending on your symptoms after those 8 weeks, your doctor will decrease the dose or discontinue the medication as needed. If your symptoms return within 3 months, your doctor will most likely recommend long-term treatment with a PPI. If your symptoms do not return within 3 months, treatment with a PPI is only needed from time to time as symptoms flare up.

If your symptoms aren't controlled with one PPI, your doctor may change your type of PPI or the dosage. In addition, further testing may be necessary to either confirm diagnosis of acid reflux, or determine if another problem is causing your symptoms. Research has repeatedly shown that the best and most effective therapy for acid reflux consists of lifestyle adjustments along with PPI.

It's important to note that hydrochloric acid (HCl) plays an important role in protecting your stomach from dangerous bacteria and pathogens, and helps with digestion. Long-term low levels of HCl—in this case induced by PPI ingestions—may result in decreased protein and vitamin digestion and may expose your gut to infections such as C. difficile. In addition, PPIs can become expensive when taken for a long time. Finding a balance between medication and other methods of treatment is a preferred method of tackling acid reflux.

The last class of medication is prokinetics. These work to help strengthen the LES and increase or strengthen the muscle contractions of the digestive tract to ultimately increase gastric emptying. This way, the contents of the stomach do not linger there, which lessens the chance of refluxing. Prokinetics are used for a variety of GI disorders but sometimes may be used for acid reflux. Medications include Urecholine (bethanechol) and Reglan (metoclopramide).

Side effects for the prokinetics include fatigue, sleepiness, depression, anxiety, and difficulty with physical movement. The side effects are often frequent, which truly limits the usefulness of the medication.

ACID ALERT

The American Gastroenterological Association Institute is against the use of certain prokinetics as a therapy for acid reflux because the side effects outweigh the benefits.

Medications That Can Hurt

Certain medications you might be taking for other ailments may make your acid reflux worse, either as a side effect or due to intolerance. Therefore, it's important for you to be aware of medications you may be on that may worsen your acid reflux symptoms. Here are some examples of medications that cause problems:

- Nonsteroidal anti-inflammatory drugs (NSAIDs) like aspirin and Aleve (also associated with an increased risk of peptic ulcers).
- Calcium channel blockers for high blood pressure or angina.
- Anticholinergics for urinary tract infections, allergies, or glaucoma.
- Beta adrenergic agonist for asthma or obstructive lung disease.
- Dopamine for Parkinson's disease.
- Bisphosphonates for osteoporosis.
- Some sedatives, antibiotics, potassium supplements, or iron pills.

Be sure to talk to your doctor about replacements for any medications that may aggravate your acid reflux.

What About Surgery?

Surgery might be an option for you if medication and lifestyle adjustments don't help alleviate your acid reflux symptoms and they interfere with your quality of life and/or have caused permanent damage to your esophagus.

Fundoplication is the standard and most effective surgical treatment for acid reflux. With this procedure, the uppermost portion of the stomach is wrapped around the LES to reinforce and to strengthen the LES. This procedure prevents acid reflux and is safe and effective for people of all ages. The most popular form is called the Nissen fundoplication. It's performed using a minimally invasive technique, leaving the patient with small incisions, less pain, a shorter hospital stay, and a higher rate of success.

Candidates for this procedure include people who have moderate to severe symptoms of GERD and wish to avoid life-long dependence on medication. If you require a medication, particularly H2 blockers, for more than a year; if you continue to suffer from the symptoms of acid reflux even though you're on the maximum dose of medication possible; if you have recurrent peptic strictures; or if you have complications of acid reflux like difficulty breathing or are at risk for aspiration, you might be a good candidate for surgery.

This procedure may increase stomach emptying and improve muscle contraction in about half of patients. About 90 percent of patients who undergo this surgery have no heartburn after the procedure. It may also cure GERD-induced respiratory problems in a significant number of patients. In general, though, complications can still occur after surgery, and you may require medication even after surgery.

Endoscopic techniques are another type of surgery but have only been used in clinical research. The long-term effects are still unknown.

The Least You Need to Know

- Lifestyle changes can greatly help in the alleviation of acid reflux symptoms.
- Quitting smoking, lowering your stress levels, getting more and better sleep, and dressing for comfort can all help reduce reflux.

- It's important to know your meds—those that can help lower your reflux symptoms and those that can make them worse.
- If all else fails, surgical intervention is an option to deal with acid reflux.

Chapter 3

Weight Management with Acid Reflux

In This Chapter

- Commonalities with acid reflux and weight
- What's considered overweight?
- Becoming a successful loser
- Take it off and keep it off

Did you know your weight might be affecting your acid reflux? If you're carrying extra pounds, especially around your midsection, you might be experiencing more acid reflux symptoms than you would if you were at a lower weight. Unfortunately, many of today's diets promote foods and behaviors that can trigger and further exacerbate your reflux symptoms. In this chapter, I share some simple pointers for deciphering whether a diet is worth your time and effort and help you develop your own acid reflux–friendly plan tailored for success.

Eating delicious, nutritious, healthy food should be an enjoyable experience. And it can be. Keep reading to learn how to achieve your weight-related goals by eating the right foods.

The Connection Between Reflux and Weight

Obesity is one of the biggest risk factors for acid reflux, erosive esophagitis, and esophageal adenocarcinoma. One study shows a significant correlation between *body mass index (BMI)* and waist circumference with lots of pressure in the stomach and esophagus.

DEFINITION

BMI (body mass index) is the relationship between weight and height that's associated with increased body fat and increased health risk. Here's the formula: body weight in kilograms ÷ height in meters, squared. A person with BMI of 25 or above is considered overweight and is at an increased risk for chronic diseases. (More on BMI later in this chapter.)

Obesity also is associated with disruption of the lower esophageal sphincter (LES), leading to hiatal hernia and increased acid exposure to the esophagus. Abdominal obesity, particularly, is associated with increased reflux symptoms. Even a moderate weight gain in women of normal weight can potentially cause a worsening of acid reflux symptoms. If you're apple-shape, you might be more at risk because the extra weight presses on your stomach and contributes to the relaxation of your LES, leading to reflux.

Although some people continue to experience symptoms even at their ideal body weight, weight loss is still recommended for obese people. It has shown very beneficial results for many acid reflux sufferers.

Are You Overweight?

The first step in managing your weight is to determine whether you are over, under, or at your ideal and healthy weight. A few standard formulas are used to asses this information. The most common one is the BMI. To calculate your BMI, first determine your weight in pounds.

Plug that number into the following formula:

$$\text{BMI} = \text{weight in pounds} \times 703 \div \text{height in inches}^2$$

Now that you have your number, here's how to interpret it:

<18.5 = underweight

18.5 to 24.9 = normal weight

25 to 29.9 = overweight

30 to 34.9 = obese class I

35 to 39.9 = obese class II

>40 = obese class III

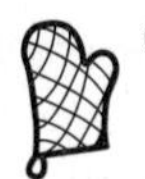

COOLER TALK

If you're a body-builder or a professional athlete, you may be frustrated with your BMI calculation. One major drawback of the BMI calculation is that it doesn't differentiate between lean muscle and fat.

Another way to determine your ideal body weight is to use the following formulas:

For women, take 100 pounds for the first 5 feet of your height and add an additional 5 pounds for each additional inch of height. To determine your ideal range, take plus or minus 10 percent from that number.

So the following would be an ideal body weight for a 5'4" female:

> 120 pounds +/– 10 percent = 108 to 132 pounds

For men, take 106 pounds for the first 5 feet of height and add an additional 6 pounds for each additional inch of height. To determine the ideal weight range, add or subtract 10 percent from this number.

For a 5'6" guy, the following would be an ideal body weight:

> 142 pounds +/– 10 percent = 128 to 156 pounds

Why such a large weight range? Because we're all built differently, and some people have much larger frames and bone structures than others.

To determine if you should be on the lower or the higher end of the spectrum, take your middle finger and your thumb, and wrap them around your wrist. If your fingers overlap, you have a small frame and should be on the lower end of the weight range. If your fingers just touch, your ideal weight is likely somewhere in the middle. If your fingers can't reach all the way around, your ideal weight is on the higher end of the range.

Setting Calorie Goals

It's important to know how many calories you need in a day. I'm not talking strict calorie counting, but you do need to know the general number of calories you need per day to help with your weight-management goals.

The simplest way to determine your calorie goals is to determine the number of calories you need per pound of body weight:

12 or 13 calories per pound for weight loss

15 or 16 calories per pound for weight maintenance

18 or 19 calories per pound for weight gain

The drawback of this method is that it doesn't account for lifestyle and activity factors.

Another way to approximate your daily intake is to calculate your basal metabolic rate (BMR). This is the number of calories you need to consume to maintain your basic body functions at rest such as breathing and circulation.

For women:

BMR = 655 + (9.6 × weight in kilograms) + (1.8 × height in centimeters) – (4.7 × age in years)

For men:

BMR = 66 + (13.7 × weight in kilograms) + (5 × height in centimeters) – (6.8 × age in years)

(To convert your weight from pound to kilograms, use this formula: 2.2 pounds = 1 kilogram. To find your height in centimeters, use this conversion: 1 inch = 2.54 centimeters.)

Because activity levels vary significantly from person to person, you'll need to multiply your BMR number by the following activity factors:

Activity Level	Men	Women
Rather inactive (sit in a chair all day)	1.4	1.4
Light daily activity	1.5	1.5
Moderately active	1.78	1.64
Very active (think professional athlete)	2.1	1.82

Remember, 1 pound of weight equals 3,500 calories. To lose 1 pound, you need to subtract that many calories through diet, exercise, or both. If you subtract 250 calories per day from your BMR through diet and another 250 through exercise, you'll have a 500-calorie deficit daily. 500 × 7 = 3,500. That equals 1 pound weight loss per week.

TUMMY TAMER

A healthy range for weight loss is 1 or 2 pounds per week. Many studies have shown that rapid weight loss above 2 pounds per week is followed by weight regain. Remember, as the pounds disappear, so will your acid reflux symptoms.

There's only one exception to these rules. No matter where these numbers fall and what your goals are, be sure to eat at least 1,200 calories per day. That's the minimum number of calories required to meet all your daily nutrient needs and keep your metabolism up.

Creating Your Best Diet

In the world of pills, shakes, bars, and meal delivery services, it may be hard to decipher which diet is the best fit for you.

Recognizing the Impostors

Here are a few red flags that tell you a diet is an impostor, one that likely won't work for you and will only lead to frustration:

- The diet promises weight loss of more than 1 or 2 pounds per week, especially after the first week or two.
- The diet eliminates one or more foods groups from your meal plan.
- The meal plan requires you to purchase expensive pills, shakes, or other ingredients.
- The diet promises weight loss without exercise. Even though this is theoretically possible, it's very unhealthy.

If you see any of these, run away. Fast!

Creating a Balanced Plan

Fortunately, creating a balanced diet that will keep you full and happy is easy! The foundation is similar for weight loss and weight maintenance. (If weight maintenance is your goal, follow these steps and incorporate one or two treat meals per week.)

First, keep all trigger foods out of your house! You know what foods I'm talking about—the ones you start eating and then can't stop. Keeping them in the house not only may be dangerous for your waistline, but overeating large quantities of foods may trigger acid reflux symptoms, too.

Incorporate a source of lean protein and fiber with every meal and snack. Protein aids with satiety and has a positive effect on acid reflux. Fiber helps with satiety and gastrointestinal function and has a slew of other health benefits. By combining these two superpowers in your meals, you'll stabilize your blood sugar levels and feel full of energy. (See Chapters 4 and 5 for good sources of fiber and protein.)

Consume 3 servings of fat-free dairy per day. If you're lactose intolerant or identify that dairy is a trigger for your acid reflux, try unsweetened almond milk and soy milk. Dairy is a good source of calcium and is very important for osteoporosis prevention. Even the nondairy alternatives are fortified, making them equivalent substitutes.

Drink plenty of water throughout the day. Your body tends to confuse thirst for hunger, which may result in overeating. Shoot for 8 to 12 (8-ounce) glasses. Drink enough throughout the day so you don't feel thirsty, a natural gauge for your body to maintain adequate hydration status.

To help get more fluids and also trick your stomach into thinking it's fuller faster, begin your restaurant meals with a broth-based soup. Studies show that people who practice this habit eat significantly less at dinner.

Use 9-inch plates when eating at home, and fill them 1/4 with protein, 1/4 with starch, and the rest with vegetables. This eliminates calorie counting and builds a perfect plate!

Load up on nonstarchy vegetables. They're your "free" foods! For only 25 calories, you can have 1/2 cup eggplant, cucumbers, okra, broccoli, mushrooms, asparagus, or many other vegetables. You'll get full way before you gain an ounce.

ACID ALERT

Alcohol is a frequent acid reflux enemy. If you decide to have a drink, stick to one or at most two drinks per day. More than that leads to increased fat accumulation and increased risk of chronic health conditions.

Exercise at least 30 minutes per day. Walking counts!

Sleep at least 7 hours per night. Sleep deprivation makes you crave fatty and sugary foods and simply leaves more hours in the day to hit the kitchen for more food. (Turn to Chapter 2 for tips on sleeping to avoid acid reflux.)

Meal Delivery Services

In the past few years, meal delivery services have been gaining popularity. Magazines report that many celebrities lose weight on them, and many patients in my practice are determined to try them.

Home-delivered meals and prepackaged foods do have some great advantages—they save you time and take the guesswork out of calorie counting. On the other hand, many of these foods are filled with acid reflux triggers such as pepper and tomato sauce.

If you decide to go this route, please read all the labels very carefully. If opting for a meal delivery service, discuss with the representative if it would be possible to alter the menus to be acid reflux friendly. Not all reps may be aware of all the possible triggers, so keep your list of triggers handy and talk details!

Planning for Long-Term Success

Some of the main reasons why diets fail are because of hunger and lack of variety. Setting unrealistic expectations is another diet downfall, as is selecting a plan that's too costly or doesn't fit into your everyday life.

Even if today is the first day of your new eating plan, it may be a good idea to start planning for long-term success sooner rather than later.

Warding Off Hunger

Many people believe hunger is a normal part of dieting. The truth is, hunger is a signal your body sends that you need to eat! Don't fight it or suppress it. Simply be sure to select lean proteins, fruits you can tolerate, and ample vegetables to satisfy your hunger pangs.

TUMMY TAMER

Fat-free Greek yogurt with 10 pistachios and 1 tablespoon honey provides a perfect combination of filling protein, healthy fats, and just the right amount of sweetness to keep you full and satisfied.

Ensuring Variety

Eating the same dishes every day may produce great short-term results, but over time, you might get bored of the same old, same old. That's a danger zone for resorting to your old favorites.

Instead, add variety and spice to your dishes by substituting slivered almonds for sesame seeds or using peanut oil instead of olive oil to awaken your taste buds. Make savory oatmeal instead of the traditional sweet version and add confectioners' sugar and cinnamon to plain popcorn to make a sweet treat. When you vary your diet, you keep your taste buds interested!

Are Your Expectations Realistic?

As noted earlier, a reasonable rate of weight loss is 1 or 2 pounds per week. The results may be faster during the first couple weeks but should stabilize by week 3 or 4.

If a week or two go by with no weight loss, don't despair! Constipation (seriously, weigh yourself before and after you go to the bathroom), excess salt consumption, and hormonal fluctuations can all contribute to the result. Be patient with yourself and stick to your plan.

Dieting on a Budget

Ideally, a diet or meal plan should be a variation on what you're already doing, taking into account your food preferences, cooking patterns, health goals, and budget. It's possible to create an exceptional meal plan on a very reasonable budget. After all, oatmeal, eggs, and beans are fairly affordable. Canned, salt-free vegetables and frozen fruits and veggies are also budget conscious.

Steer clear of the diets that ask you to purchase expensive ingredients. Maybe use that money to invest in a gym membership instead!

Does the Plan Fit Your Lifestyle?

Opting for a plan that doesn't fit your lifestyle is the equivalent of setting yourself up for failure. For example, if you order a meal delivery service when you enjoy eating out on a nightly basis, you'll likely not use the delivered food, wasting it and your money.

Instead, if you eat out and entertain, determine ways to stay on track by identifying the best dishes on the restaurant menus. If cooking for four kids on a nightly basis is a must, find recipes that can work for your entire family.

Whatever you do, work *with* your lifestyle, not *against* it.

TUMMY TAMER

If you have a hard time devising a balanced plan yourself, find a registered dietitian who can help. Many dietitians accept insurance and can be a great asset in guiding you toward your goals. Visit eatright.org to find a dietitian near you.

Lapse Versus Relapse

You're only human, and putting the words *always* and *never* in your sentences may set you up for failure.

As most experienced dieters and people who maintain long-term weight loss results will tell you, lapses happen. Temptations at birthday parties, dinners out with clients, or an extra donut left over by your spouse may all bring back the old habits. To succeed, make a specific plan of action you can execute just in case a lapse occurs.

Your first step should be to get right back on track with the next meal instead of the next day. Your next bite counts!

Also, don't skip meals to compensate for the lapse. Instead, head over to the gym for an extra hour of training and include low-sodium foods full of protein and fiber combined with ample water to make you feel better.

If the scale is your gauge, staying within 5 pounds of your ideal body weight is a great goal. If your scale creeps up by 1 or 2 pounds, you might attribute it to water retention or constipation. When your pants get tight and you're gaining more than 5 pounds, it may be time to re-examine your diet.

The Least You Need to Know

- The body mass index is a good way to evaluate whether you're overweight.
- Setting realistic weight management expectations is the first step to success in managing both your weight and your acid reflux symptoms.
- Regardless of your goal, aim to create a balanced meal plan using unprocessed natural foods that don't trigger your reflux.
- Select a strategy that best fits into your life and helps keep your acid reflux at bay, and plan for long-term success at the get go.
- Prepare for possible lapses and have a plan of action that can be executed at this time.

Ensuring Your Success on the Acid Reflux Diet

Part

2

Eating well and acid reflux control are not mutually exclusive. Your diet should consist of the right amount of protein, carbohydrates, and fats to keep your body functioning properly and controlling reflux symptoms. But what's the right amount? Part 2 delves into the proteins, carbohydrates, and fats you need, along with their functions, their connection to the reflux symptoms, and the appropriate amount for your diet.

To help you put all this into practice, I also include a chapter on meal planning and supermarket shopping tips, complete with sample meal ideas.

I wrap up Part 2 with a chapter on exercise. In it, I tell you the worst and best exercises you can do to control acid reflux, and I help you find great snacks and meals to power through your workouts.

Chapter 4

Fats and Proteins

In This Chapter

- The connection between fat and acid reflux
- Fats: good and bad
- Understanding your fat needs
- Protein's influence on acid reflux
- Getting enough protein

Every day, you breathe, eat, move, and attend to a host of activities. To do all those things, you need energy, and that energy comes from the food you eat. Food provides the energy, measured in calories, you need to keep up with life. The calories are used in your body like fuel in a car.

Food can be categorized into three different macronutrients: fat, protein, and carbohydrates. (They're called *macronutrients* because your body uses them in large amounts.) All three macronutrients are equally important for your body to function properly. We take a closer look at fat and protein in this chapter and save carbohydrates for Chapter 5.

These macronutrients can contain micronutrients, which your body only needs in small amounts. Even though you only require small amounts, micronutrients pack a big punch. They help produce enzymes, hormones, and other substances that help your body grow and develop properly at every stage of life. Micronutrients consist mainly of vitamins and minerals.

The Skinny on Fat

Fat is the most calorie-dense macronutrient, meaning it has more calories per gram than protein and carbohydrates do. Fat has 9 kilocalories per gram, while protein and carbohydrates both have 4 kilocalories per gram.

Fat serves different functions. Fat from your diet, for example, is stored in your fat cells. Your body is able to store and use large amounts of fat, which is important for survival in times of famine. Structural fat holds organs and nerves in place and protects your body from injury, shock, or pressure. Subcutaneous fat, found below your skin, insulates your body for heat and maintains body temperature.

Dietary fat is important for your body to digest, absorb, and transport fat-soluble vitamins and minerals. Dietary fat also slows down stomach-emptying so foods higher in fat linger longer in your stomach.

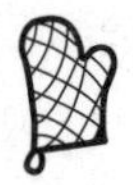

COOLER TALK

Although you might not think of alcohol as containing fat, it does contain calories—7 calories per gram, and with no nutritional value. That's why alcohol is often referred to as a source of empty calories.

We are "hardwired" to prefer the taste of fat because fat is necessary to survive. For example, people tend to enjoy the taste and texture of high-fat chocolate more than fat-free chocolate. Fat is often used in cooking for the texture, smoothness, tenderness, and feelings of fullness after a meal it provides.

While it might be natural to crave fat, you still should be smart with your fat choices. Fat is higher in calories than the other two macronutrients, so it's essential to choose healthier types of fat. Also, only have fat in moderation to prevent weight gain and symptoms of acid reflux. For instance, heart-healthy fats such as avocados and olive oil are healthy when consumed in moderation. The added benefit of fat is that it helps you stay full longer, which means less temptation for extra calories in between meals.

Fat and Acid Reflux

Fat affects acid reflux. Because one of the main functions of fat is delayed stomach emptying, fatty food stays in your stomach longer. When your stomach notices food is hanging out there, it makes more acid to digest it. Fat may also decrease the lower esophageal sphincter (LES) pressure and increase relaxation of the LES.

Some studies that examine the effect of dietary fat on acid reflux have suggested that the more fat eaten during a meal, the worse the acid reflux—and even more so if the person is overweight or obese. The link is still unclear, however, and researchers are continuing to look into this theory. Other studies report that the overall caloric density of the diet, not the fat content, contributes to acid reflux.

The bottom line is that both high-fat food choices and high-calorie selections may lead to a greater risk for acid reflux.

Good Fat Versus Bad Fat

Fat comes in different types. "Good" fats, if eaten in moderation, can provide total body benefits. "Bad" fats, on the other hand, can cause significant harm to the body. So it's important to choose your fats wisely. And only eat the good ones—and in moderation—because as mentioned, excess fat can intensify acid reflux.

Let's go over some of the different types of fat so you know which ones to eat and which to avoid.

Monounsaturated Fats

Monounsaturated fats, the first of the "good" fats, are simple fats that are usually in liquid form at room temperature. Foods containing these fats include vegetable oils like olive, canola, high oleic safflower, and sunflower; avocados; peanut butter; nuts; and seeds.

Replacing the bad fats in your diet (more on these coming up) with good, monounsaturated fats may decrease your low-density lipoprotein (LDL) cholesterol, the type of cholesterol you want to keep as low as possible to prevent diseases; lower your triglycerides; and maintain your high-density lipoprotein (HDL) cholesterol—the good cholesterol. Monounsaturated fats may protect against heart disease, too.

ACID ALERT

If LDL cholesterol is too high, it can increase your risk of cardiovascular disease. Your chances of getting type 2 diabetes increase, too.

Polyunsaturated Fats

Polyunsaturated fats are also simple fats typically liquid at room temperature. Foods high in polyunsaturated fats include vegetable oils like soybean, corn, and safflower; fatty fish like salmon, mackerel, herring, and trout; and some nuts and seeds like walnuts and sunflower.

Polyunsaturated fats are divided into two types: omega-3 and omega-6. You need to keep the ratio of these two "omegas" in good balance to receive the benefits of the omega-3s. The American diet is high in processed and packaged foods and, therefore, omega-6s, so it's important to consciously supplement omega-3s to maintain this balance and reap the health benefits. Omega-6s include soybean oil, corn oil, and safflower oil. Omega-3s include soybean oil, canola oil, walnuts, flaxseeds, and fish such as trout, herring, and salmon. Omega-3 is an essential nutrient, which means your body cannot produce it so you have to supply it from outside sources.

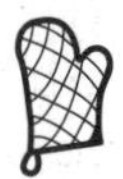

COOLER TALK

Omega-3s have several types. EPA and DHA are particularly important ones essential for health. Most omega-3 supplements include these in the nutrition label. EPA and DHA are primarily found in fish oils. Another type, ALA, is found in plant sources such as flaxseed. ALA is converted into DHA and EPA in the body.

Even if you're trying to monitor the amount of fat you consume, particularly due to acid reflux, it's still important to incorporate moderate amounts of good fats in your diet. Omega-6s from oils tend to lower LDL and HDL cholesterol, ultimately lowering the risk of heart disease. Populations with high omega-3 intake have lower rates of heart disease.

Saturated Fat

Saturated fat is not a good fat. It has earned its well-deserved bad reputation because it raises total blood cholesterol levels and LDL cholesterol (the bad cholesterol). Typically, it's solid at room temperature—think of the butter on the potato or the visible fat on the rib eye. Saturated fat comes mainly from animal sources, like fatty meats, whole milk, cheeses, egg yolks, lard, and butter.

TUMMY TAMER

A balanced diet should consist of 20 to 35 percent of total daily calories coming from fat, with 10 percent at most coming from saturated food sources. If you have acid reflux, adhere to the lower end of the recommended intake.

If you make a conscious effort to decrease your saturated fat intake—which you should, starting now—you'll also decrease your acid reflux symptoms. (As a bonus, you'll lower your chances of getting coronary heart disease and certain cancers.) Studies have shown over and over again that saturated fats are the main culprit in acid reflux, so start reading your nutrition facts label and stop eating this unfriendly fat.

Trans Fat

Trans fat is another one worth paying attention to. It's very harmful to your heart, increases LDL, and decreases HDL. This fat can occur naturally in some foods, especially animal-based foods. However, most trans fats are manmade and processed. Food scientists add an extra hydrogen into a good type of fat and make it bad. Why the added hydrogen? Because it makes the food easier to cook with and increases its shelf life. You can find trans fat in baked goods and packaged products that do not have an expiration date.

The words *partially hydrogenated* in ingredient lists indicate the presence of trans fat in the product. Once you start looking for those words, you'll find them in so many places. Trans fats and saturated fats in general should be limited because those are the ones that exacerbate acid reflux the most. Given that your fat consumption should be limited in the first place, stick to mono and polyunsaturated fats such as olive oil and avocados, and be on the lookout for the "partially hydrogenated" kind.

ACID ALERT

Manufacturers are allowed to label products "0 trans fat" as long as the product has 0.5 grams or less trans fat per serving. Many manufacturers are now increasing the number of portions so they can list a lower amount of trans fat per serving. Be sure to read and understand food labels!

How Much Fat Do You Need?

Fat is essential for survival. Although some studies have found saturated fat to be the main culprit, current thought says that regardless of the type of fat, the overall amount of fat consumed plays a role in acid reflux. High-fat meals may exacerbate symptoms, so the key is eating modest amounts of healthy fats.

The U.S. Department of Agriculture (USDA) recommends that 20 to 35 percent of your total daily calories come from fat. To avoid eating too much acid reflux–unfriendly fat, it's best to stay on the lower end of that range. But don't try to completely eliminate fat from your diet because you need some to survive and function normally.

The next time you're selecting what to eat, keep in mind these tips to help monitor your fat intake:

- Replace animal fats (saturated fat) and hydrogenated fat (trans fat) with fruits, vegetables, legumes, and whole grains.
- Decrease your saturated fat intake by replacing whole or 2 percent milk with skim or 1 percent milk.
- Avoid trans fats by staying away from stick margarine, and avoid eating commercially baked goods and deep-fried fast foods.
- When you cook with fat, stick to monounsaturated and polyunsaturated fats, especially ones with omega-3s like olive oil.
- When snacking on nuts or seeds, eat them in moderate amounts.

If you're tempted to eat a high-fat meal, be sure the portion size is less than 4 ounces—smaller than the size of your palm. Smaller portion sizes decrease the amount of acid released by your stomach. (Stay tuned for more on portion control.)

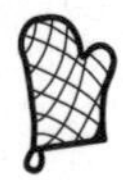

COOLER TALK

One pistachio contains about 4 calories. That means you can have 25 pistachios for 100 calories!

How can you tell what foods are high in fat? High-fat foods are generally marbled red meat like prime cuts of steak, ground beef, processed chicken products, chicken with skin on, pork ribs, roast, and lamb. Chocolate, potato or corn chips, high-fat baked goods, and creamy or oily salad dressing also fall into this category. Regular-fat-content dairy products like sour cream, milkshakes, ice cream, cottage cheese, regular-fat cheese, butter, creams, half-and-half, and cream-based soups are on the list, too. Foods made with butter like chicken Kiev, shrimp scampi, and croissants are also no-nos.

Sometimes fat is hidden in food, so you need to check food labels carefully. Nondairy creamers, gravies, sauces, and creamy soups are excellent sources of hidden fat. Frozen dinners and fried foods need lots of fat to keep them shelf stable and delicious, so beware of those. Foods low in sodium use more sugar or fat to enhance flavor. The next time you see any of these items on a menu, take a second and ask yourself if heartburn is worth the taste of these foods.

A Protein Primer

Protein plays a special role in your body because it helps with growth and repair of bodily tissues. Protein is also important for immune function and production of hormones and enzymes. This macronutrient also provides energy when carbohydrates (the preferred source of fuel) aren't available, preserving lean body mass.

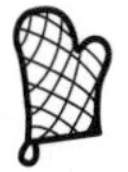

COOLER TALK

The word *protein* was mentioned in scientific publications as early as 1838. In Greek, the word means "first in rank," implying its importance.

Food made of protein is broken down to amino acids, the building blocks of protein. Some amino acids are essential, which means your body cannot make them. Protein from animal sources such as fish, dairy, poultry, and eggs contains all the essential amino acids we need, making it a complete protein. Our bodies are able to absorb almost 100 percent of protein found in those foods. Plant proteins do not have all the essential amino acids, so eating a variety of these incomplete proteins together is often recommended to ensure adequate protein intake.

Protein and Acid Reflux

Protein is recommended to help reduce incidences of acid reflux. Protein may help strengthen the LES over time, so it can function properly by serving as a barrier between the esophagus and the stomach.

Many sources of protein come from animals, like red meat, poultry, and dairy, and can be high in saturated fat. In those cases, the protein may not be as beneficial. It's best to choose lean cuts of meat and poultry with the visible fat trimmed off. Fish usually has less saturated fat than meat or poultry. When choosing dairy products, always go for the low-fat or nonfat varieties.

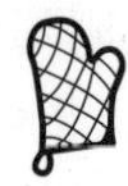

COOLER TALK

Some people drink regular milk before bedtime for relief from acid reflux. This is only a temporary fix, however, and might produce more problems later in the night because of a rebound action. Some say that drinking skim milk, if medicine is not available, helps. Skim milk has no fat, so there are no culprits to stimulate acid reflux. If you opt for skim milk for relief, only drink a small amount, and sit upright for at least 30 minutes before you move around.

Some studies have shown that certain amino acids in protein have been beneficial toward acid reflux symptoms. Glutamine, for example, may decrease the amount of inflammation in the esophagus caused by recurrent exposure to acid. Glutamine can be found in fish, chicken, beans, and eggs.

How Much Protein Do I Need?

The USDA recommends 10 to 35 percent of your calories each day should come from protein. People who are experiencing acid reflux should stick with the higher end of the range.

Another recommendation for protein intake published by the Institute of Medicine recommends 0.4 gram protein per pound per day, at minimum, for adults. A general guideline when preparing meals is to eat at least 4 ounces high-quality protein for lunch and again for dinner.

Great Protein Choices

Let's look at some of the best protein sources for the type of protein eater you may be.

TUMMY TAMER

How you cook your food can make as much of a difference as what you're cooking. The best way to prepare protein items is with low-fat methods such as grilling, broiling, stir-fry, or steaming with very little amounts of vegetable fat. Avoid frying foods unless you want to set off your acid reflux.

Omnivores

Omnivores have several choices when it comes to protein. Chicken and turkey are lower in saturated fat, and light meat is always a better choice than dark meat. Opt for skinless and boneless varieties. Chicken breast and lean turkey are great, low-fat choices:

- Chicken breast (boneless, skinless): 3.5 ounces contains 30 grams protein
- Turkey: 1 ounce contains 7 grams protein

Fish is a heart-healthy choice and an excellent source of protein, lowest in saturated fat and high in heart-healthy unsaturated fats compared to other meats. Choose orange roughy, Chilean sea bass, red snapper, grouper, and farmed salmon. Fish high in omega-3 fatty acids include wild Alaskan salmon, sockeye salmon, coho salmon, Atlantic mackerel, herring, and sardines. Other good sources of seafood include ocean perch, canned light tuna, Pacific cod, farmed tilapia, farmed catfish, farmed rainbow trout, farmed oysters, and shrimp.

From the macronutrient standpoint, 6 ounces tuna contains 40 grams protein, and 3.5 ounces salmon contains 27 grams protein. On average 3.5 ounces fish contains about 25 to 30 grams protein.

Avoid tilefish, king mackerel, swordfish, and shark. These are high in mercury.

Limit your intake of beef, pork, and lamb to less than 18 ounces per week because they are high in saturated fat. When eating these foods, try to select the loin cut. Pasture-raised or grass-fed choices seem to be healthier (and better for the environment, too). Processed red meats such as bacon, hot dogs, and deli meats are linked with higher rates of cancer. Avoid them.

Vegetarians

Vegetarians sometimes wonder how they can get adequate protein if they don't eat poultry or fish. Never fear! You have several great acid reflux–friendly foods to choose from:

- Eggs: 1 large contains 7 grams protein.
- Egg substitute: ¼ cup contains 8 grams protein.
- Milk (skim): 1 cup contains 8 grams protein.

- Cottage cheese: $^1/_2$ cup contains 15 grams protein.
- Yogurt (nonfat): 1 cup contains 8 to 12 grams protein. Greek yogurt contains 12 grams or more per cup, so that's another great option. Stick to the nonfat kind.

Egg whites are an excellent source of protein. The yolk contains all the saturated fat and cholesterol, so stick with the whites to avoid acid reflux. And because cheeses are usually high in fat, they're never a good option.

ACID ALERT

When flavoring your food, be careful with spices, peppers, onions, and chiles. They can trigger acid reflux.

Note that eating a vegetarian diet makes you more prone to vitamin deficiencies, specifically vitamin B_{12}, calcium, iron, and zinc. It's important that you find out from your doctor whether you are or are not deficient in these vitamins or minerals. Some acid reflux medications neutralize the acid in your stomach to alleviate reflux symptoms. One of the major functions of the acid is to help absorb vitamins and minerals. With excessive use of these medications, over time, you can develop deficiencies that can lead to serious health complications.

Vegans

I haven't forgotten you, vegans! Nuts and seeds contain lots of fat, but mostly the heart-healthy type, so consume these in moderation for a great source of vegan protein. Nuts that contain less than 2 grams saturated fat per ounce include almonds, chestnuts, hazelnuts, pecans, peanuts, pistachios, and walnuts. Nuts and seeds that have more than 2 grams saturated fat per ounce are Brazil nuts, cashews, macadamia nuts, and coconuts, so limit the latter.

Beans, soy products, and whole grains are also on your good-protein list. Beans are heart healthy and are good sources of protein, fiber, and healthy carbohydrates. Soy products and tofu contain fat, so pick low-fat varieties when available. Whole grains like quinoa are an excellent source of protein and fiber. They're the most complete plant protein, and they're low in fat.

Here are some great protein choices for vegans:

- Almonds, peanuts, and cashews: $\frac{1}{4}$ cup contains 8, 9, and 5 grams protein, respectively.
- Peanut butter: 2 tablespoons contain 8 grams protein.
- Beans: 6 to 10 grams fiber and 6 to 8 grams protein in $\frac{1}{2}$ cup.
- Soybeans: $\frac{1}{2}$ cup contains 11 grams protein.
- Tofu (firm): $\frac{1}{2}$ cup contains 2 grams protein.
- Soy milk: 1 cup contains 11 grams protein.
- Vegetable or soy patty: 1 patty contains 11 grams protein.
- Whole grains like quinoa: 1 cup contains 4 to 6 grams fiber and 7 to 9 grams protein.

ACID ALERT

Soy and tofu products can be naturally high in fat or loaded with extra fat and calories due to the preparation method. Opt for low-fat varieties whenever possible.

Increase your bean and soy products to meet adequate protein and essential amino acid intake. Also, it's recommended that vegans increase their protein consumption by 25 percent if they rely mainly on beans or foods with low digestibility.

Protein Powders and Supplements

The majority of protein in your diet should be supplied from whole foods. Natural foods are packed with fiber, vitamins, and minerals. Protein supplements can be a quick and convenient method of increasing protein only if you're significantly lacking it in your diet.

Even the most muscular bodybuilders only need 1.2 to 1.7 grams protein per kilogram body weight per day. That means a 220-pound man requires between 120 and 170 grams protein per day. Sixteen ounces of milk contain 16 grams protein, a 3.5-ounce chicken breast has 30 grams, and a 6-ounce can of tuna has 39 grams. Even 1 cup whole-wheat pasta contains 7.5 grams protein. See how easy it is to meet the daily protein requirement just by consuming natural foods?

Now, if you're no body builder and are instead a moderately active 150-pound female, you only require 0.8 to 1 gram protein per kilogram of body weight, or 54 to 68 grams protein. If you eat a well-balanced diet, it's highly unlikely you'll need protein supplements.

Other options in lieu of protein supplements include boosting recipes or foods with other foods high in protein. You could add dried milk to foods or use nonfat or low-fat milk instead of water in recipes. Try adding cottage cheese to your fruit. Mix hard-boiled eggs without the yolk with meat, tuna, salads, sauces, and casseroles. You also can add yogurt as a snack or a dressing to fruit.

TUMMY TAMER

To convert from pounds to kilograms, divide the weight in pounds by 2.2.

If you're convinced you need to supplement, it's important to educate yourself before choosing one. Different types of protein supplements are available.

Avoid concentrated soy protein or extracts like isoflavones. The long-term effects are still unknown.

Whey protein is a good choice for supplementing protein. Because whey comes from milk, the protein powder is a high-quality, complete protein, containing all amino acids. Whey protein is typically low in fat and carbohydrates. Whey protein isolate is the leanest type of whey. Whey protein concentrate contains more fat and carbohydrate, and it's less expensive than whey protein isolate. The choice is yours, but either protein is a good option because these proteins are similar in their biological effects on the body.

Meal replacement powders are a blend of different protein types and contain both fat and carbohydrates, so their contents are similar to eating a meal. If you're watching your fat consumption, meal replacement powders may not be the best sources of protein.

ACID ALERT

Many protein powders and meal replacement products contain artificial sweeteners that may exacerbate acid reflux.

When searching for supplements, be aware of what you're buying. Manufacturers of dietary supplements can't legally say their product can diagnose, cure, treat, or prevent disease. They can say their supplement contributes to health maintenance and well-being.

The U.S. Food and Drug Administration (FDA) does not regulate dietary supplements the same way it regulates medicine, and dietary supplements can be sold without researching how well they work. The FDA states that the dietary supplement manufacturer is responsible for the safety of the supplement before it hits the market, but manufacturers do not need to register their products with the FDA or get FDA approval. They must, however, be sure the information on the product is not misleading. Once the product has hit the market, the FDA will then monitor the safety.

U.S. Pharmacopeia (USP) is a verification program that ensures manufacturers, regulatory authorities, and consumers get assurances that drug substances with the USP Verified Mark are of consistent ingredients and high quality. USP establishes standards for medicine, food ingredients, and dietary supplement products and ingredients. USP ingredient verification helps companies reach best-quality management and provides drug substance manufacturers with Good Manufacturing Practices with auditing, review, laboratory testing, reporting, and surveillance. For more information, visit usp.org.

The Least You Need to Know

- If you reduce trans and saturated fats in your diet, you reduce your chances of an acid reflux flare-up.
- Including healthy sources of fats such as nuts, olive oil, and avocado in small amounts helps you reduce cholesterol and supply your body with much needed omega-3s and omega-6s. Think teaspoons.
- Incorporating lean protein with your meals can help reduce acid reflux symptoms.
- Avoid protein powders unless absolutely necessary in a state of deficiency or malnutrition.

Chapter

5

Carbohydrates

In This Chapter

- All about carbohydrates
- Fiber basics
- How carbs and fiber affect reflux
- Types and sources of fiber

Carbohydrates have gained an unfortunate bad rep due to all the low-carb weight-loss diets hitting the market within the last few decades. The truth is, our bodies need carbohydrates, just as they do protein and fat, to function properly.

Not all carbohydrates are created equally, however, and some are better than others. In this chapter, I give you the tools you need to select the best types of carbohydrates for reducing acid reflux symptoms and improving your overall health.

Fiber is a type of carbohydrate and is an important nutrient to have. Your body can't digest it, so it passes through your digestive system, absorbing unhelpful nutrients and eliminating waste. Fiber has so many potential health benefits that it's considered a wonder food.

Carbohydrate Basics

Carbohydrates are the preferred source of energy for your brain, and you need this macronutrient in larger quantities than fat or protein. Foods high in carbohydrates are broken down into glucose, an important source of energy for all tissues and cells. Carbohydrates are necessary for your central nervous system to function, too. Your brain, muscles, and heart would not function at peak capacity without carbs.

Carbohydrates can be stored in your muscles and liver to be used for energy later when it's not readily available. Carbohydrates also are important for intestinal health and waste elimination. That's a lot for one nutrient to do!

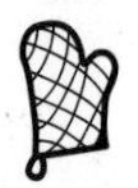

COOLER TALK

Your brain needs 5 grams carbohydrates per hour to function normally.

Carbohydrates are mainly found in starchy foods like grains, fruits, milk, and yogurt. You can also find them in sugary products like cakes, cookies, and sugar-sweetened beverages such as soda and fruit juices.

As you can probably imagine, not all carbohydrates are created equally. When choosing foods, pick those that contain "complex carbohydrates." It takes your body longer to digest these carbs, and they provide energy for a longer time. So you can eat less of these foods while feeling fuller for a longer time. Complex carbs are loaded in vitamins, minerals, and other micronutrients that do wonders in your body. Examples of complex carbohydrates include whole grains, beans and legumes, and sweet potatoes.

Avoid "simple carbohydrates" such as cakes, cookies, sodas, and sweetened products. They're considered bad carbohydrates because they're easily digested and offer no vitamin or mineral benefits. Plus, they can easily lead to weight gain if eaten in excess. Eating foods high in simple sugars often makes you crave more—it's a vicious cycle.

Be picky with your carbohydrates! Opt for the ones that benefit your body and make you a healthy, vibrant person.

Fantastic Fiber

The benefits of a diet rich in fiber are endless. Fiber is a fantastic health food, especially when you get it from whole foods, those foods not processed and as close to natural as you can get. Think whole grains, fruits, and vegetables.

Fiber comes in two forms: soluble and insoluble.

Soluble fiber is made of carbohydrates and easily dissolves in water. Once soluble fiber hits your intestines, it begins to absorb water and comes to a gel-like consistency. This gel helps push food slowly and smoothly through your gut to make you feel fuller longer. Along with the water, it absorbs cholesterol and bad substances and helps eliminate it via stool. Soluble fiber helps prevent high blood cholesterol and high blood sugars. Examples include fruits, oats, nuts, barley, flax, and legumes.

Insoluble fiber has a slightly different function from soluble fiber. Found in plant cell walls, it does not dissolve in water like soluble fiber. However, it does help move food quickly through the digestive tract, removing toxic waste in the intestines and decreasing its exposure time in the colon. Insoluble fiber also adds bulk to stool, helps prevent constipation, and helps keep an overall healthy bowel. Examples include vegetables such as green beans and dark-green leafy vegetables, root vegetable skins, fruit, whole-wheat items, nuts, and seeds.

TUMMY TAMER

If you have acid reflux, try grains. They're good for you, and you should be able to tolerate them well. However, do pay attention to the method of preparation, and avoid those high in fat and prepared with tomato sauce. Macaroni and cheese or pasta with marinara or heavy cream sauce, for example, could trigger your symptoms.

Carbohydrates, Fiber, and Reflux

Luckily, good carbs like complex carbs are beneficial for your acid reflux. Fiber is a very complex carbohydrate that offers many health benefits. Most dietary fiber is not digested or absorbed, so it stays in your intestines longer, helping with the digestion of other foods and also waste elimination.

Choosing fiber from the right sources can help your acid reflux. Fiber-rich foods help eliminate food faster and remove toxins from the body. This way, substances spend a shorter amount of time in the intestinal tract, preventing gastrointestinal issues that can lead to acid reflux. It's thought that bacteria in the intestinal tract may produce different by-products high in acid. If the fiber doesn't clean up these bacteria and absorb them for elimination, unwanted acid reflux can occur.

Some studies have shown that a high-fiber diet is associated with a decreased risk of reflux. Adding even 1 gram fiber to your diet a day is associated with a decreased risk of recurrent and frequent reflux. It's that easy. Add 1 serving of a fruit or vegetable to your diet each day, and you'll feel a huge improvement in your reflux symptoms.

Fiber also helps neutralize the stomach's acidic environment. When you eat certain foods, their by-products linger in the stomach until they're ready to move into the intestines. Some of these substances have a potential to relax the lower esophageal sphincter (LES), which promotes reflux. Fiber has been shown to absorb these substances in the stomach, decreasing the chances of these substances affecting the LES and preventing reflux episodes.

It's important to note that although fiber is shown to have a tremendous effect on reducing reflux, you should avoid soluble fiber that comes from citrus fruits and tomatoes. Those could trigger acid reflux.

ACID ALERT

Oranges, grapefruits, lemons, limes, cranberries, and tomatoes are all amazing super foods. If you have acid reflux, they may also be your enemies. Steer clear of these foods, or introduce one at a time in very small amounts and monitor your tolerance.

How Much Carbs and Fiber Do You Need?

The USDA's Dietary Reference Intakes (DRI) recommend that 45 to 65 percent of your total calories per day should come from carbohydrates. Fiber is about 25 grams per day for women and 30 grams per day for men.

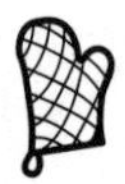

COOLER TALK

RDI (Recommended Daily Intake) is the daily intake of a certain nutrient you need to meet the 97 to 98 percent of the population in every demographic. Don't confuse it with DRI (Dietary Reference Intake), which is a system of nutrition recommendations from Institute of Medicine and a general term for accepted dietary values for healthy people. These values vary by gender and age.

The following table lists some good sources of fiber you can include in your acid reflux–friendly diet.

Food	Serving	Grams Fiber
Starches:		
Bagel, whole-wheat	¼ large	1.5
Bran muffin	1 medium	5.2

Food	Serving	Grams Fiber
Bread, whole-wheat	1 slice	3
Bulgur, cooked	½ cup	4.1
Cereals, whole-grain	1 cup	3.5
Corn, fresh	½ cup	4.2
English muffin	½ muffin	2.2
Oat bran	½ cup	3.5
Popcorn	3 cups	3.5
Potato, regular with skin	1 medium	3.8
Potato, sweet	½ cup mashed	3.3
Quinoa	⅓ cup	3.6
Rice, brown	1 cup	3.5
Waffle, whole-grain	1 waffle	4
Fruits:		
Apple	1 medium	3.3
Apricots	2 medium	1.4
Banana	1 small	2.1
Blackberries	¾ cup	5.7
Blueberries	¾ cup	2.6
Cantaloupe	⅓ melon	1.2
Mangoes	1 small	3
Nectarines	1 small	2.2
Papaya	1 cup	1.3
Raspberries	1 cup	8
Strawberries	1 cup	3.3
Vegetables:		
Asparagus	1 cup raw	1.8
Beets	1 cup raw	1.7
Broccoli	1 cup raw	2.6
Carrots, sliced	½ cup raw	2.3
Cauliflower	1 cup raw	2.5
Eggplant	1 cup raw	2.8
Hearts of palm	1 cup raw	4.3
Swiss chard	1 cup raw	1.8
Turnips	1 cup raw	2.3

continues

continued

Food	Serving	Grams Fiber
Legumes:		
Baked beans, canned	1 cup	13.9
Kidney beans, canned	1 cup	13.6
Lentils, boiled	1 cup	15.6
Lima beans, canned	1 cup	11.6
Nuts and nut butters:		
Almonds	1 ounce	3.3
Cashews	1 ounce	0.9
Nut butters	1 tablespoon	~1
Peanuts	1 ounce	2.3
Pistachios	1 ounce	2.9

Tips for Getting More Fiber

If you eat a diet high in whole foods—foods as close to nature as possible and not highly processed—you may be getting the fiber you need. However, eating processed foods such as white bread and rice and an overall "Americanized" diet can make it very difficult to get the recommended amount of fiber you need in your diet.

Here are some tips that can get you to where you need to be fiber wise:

- Be sure to eat whole grains, especially bread and cereal. Look for 100 percent whole wheat, rye, oats, or bran as the first or second ingredient in the ingredients list.
- Eat protein-packed brown or wild rice instead of white rice or potato.
- Enjoy a variety of grains such as barley, oats, farro, kamut, and quinoa.
- Choose fruits and vegetables—with their peels and skins on—over fruit and vegetable juices.

When you add fiber to your diet, remember to drink more water with it. If you don't drink enough water, you may be at risk for constipation.

What About Fiber Supplements?

Many fiber supplements are on the market these days. Generally, supplements are not recommended. Instead, it's best to get your fiber through whole foods found as close to nature as possible. As a bonus, these foods come with super-powered vitamins, minerals, and antioxidants, too. Plus real food tastes better! Just a few servings of fiber-rich foods can help you meet your fiber needs.

Supplements, in general, are safe. However, as previously mentioned, you must drink plenty of water when taking fiber supplements to ward off possible constipation. Psyllium is one fiber supplement that absorbs water and expands in the intestine. It can cause bloating and is not ideal for long-term use. However, Metamucil (the brand name of psyllium) is bulk forming and can be used as a laxative for constipation. Konsyl is another type of psyllium. It contains more fiber than Metamucil or Benefiber and helps with constipation.

Methylcellulose, also known as Citrucel, or "smart fiber," does not cause excess gas or bloating like psyllium. It's not used to treat constipation because it's not a laxative, but it does promote regularity. Wheat dextrin, also known as Benefiber, does not contain psyllium or inulin. It's a natural form of soluble fiber that can be mixed or dissolved into foods.

It's recommended that you start to supplement with a small amount and slowly increase until stool becomes softer and more frequent.

Bottom line: supplements are generally expensive, so if you're healthy and have a well-balanced diet, they may not be worth the cost.

The Least You Need to Know

- Carbohydrates are a necessary part of a well-balanced diet.
- Dietary fiber is your friend and helps alleviate acid reflux symptoms.
- Fiber supplements are safe, but it's always better to meet your daily fiber goals through natural food choices instead.

Chapter 6

Menu Planning and Smart Shopping Strategies

In This Chapter

- A look at the acute phase reflux diet
- How to control chronic symptoms
- Keeping a food journal
- Supermarket shopping essentials

By now you know that too much fat may trigger your reflux symptoms and that protein and fiber can be allies in your fight against acid reflux. However, the game of managing acid reflux is not that simple. You need to be aware of what foods are acid reflux friendly and what foods are not.

This chapter gives you the tools you need to create a specific diet customized to your current symptoms. A guide to supermarket shopping further ensures you have all the information necessary for creating a well-balanced meal plan that's free of acid reflux triggers.

The Acute Phase Diet

The term *acute* refers to a time when you're experiencing severe symptoms. During that period, it's best to start with the strictest dietary regimen possible, weeding out potentially harmful foods until you feel better. At that point, you may consider reintroducing certain foods and food combinations one at a time to determine how you respond to them.

What to Eat, What Not to Eat

During the acute stage, avoid the following:

- Citrus fruits and juices
- Products that contain vinegar such as dressings
- Tomatoes and tomato-based products
- Onions and garlic
- Leeks
- Spicy foods
- Pepper
- Ketchup and mustard
- High-fat foods (even the good type of fat)
- Chocolate
- Mint and peppermint
- Alcohol (all types)
- Carbonated beverages
- Coffee

In addition to fried foods such as onion rings and french fries, stay away from other high-fat foods like mashed potatoes, potato salad, macaroni and cheese, pastas with heavy cream sauces, and cream-based soups. Even healthy fats in large amounts may trigger acid reflux symptoms.

Instead, incorporate the following into your meal plan:

- Breads, cereals, grains, and other starches high in fiber and prepared without added fat.
- Bananas and applesauce.
- Vegetables—as long as they're prepared without extra added fat. Some people report tolerating cooked vegetables better than raw ones.
- Lean poultry and lean cuts of meat.

- Any kind of fish. Even canned varieties are great as long as they're canned in water and not oil.
- Beans prepared without added fat or spices.
- Fat-free dairy such as milk and plain yogurt. Flavored yogurts may have added chemicals that could trigger reflux symptoms. Purchase plain and flavor it yourself.
- Very small amounts of nuts and natural nut butters.
- Plain water and herbal caffeine-free teas such as chamomile. (Many herbal teas are flavored with artificial chemicals and ingredients and may provoke acid reflux symptoms. Opt for the least processed varieties. Look for organic and the least amount of ingredients in the ingredient section of the label.)
- Herbs for flavoring. (See Chapter 8 for a list of acid reflux–friendly herbs.)

Some studies report increased acid production when consuming dairy products. Contrary to these reports, many patients report symptom improvement when switching to fat-free dairy products. Keep track of how you feel to identify your tolerances.

In addition to opting for the correct food choices, meal patterns also matter. The following are some behavioral modifications you can implement to help control your acid reflux symptoms:

- Consume structured, small meals throughout the day instead of one or two large ones.

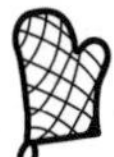

COOLER TALK

The more your stomach is stretched by food, the more likely you are to experience reflux. Smaller meals and smaller portion sizes, eaten more frequently throughout the day, keep your stomach from getting too full at any given point. A too-full stomach increases production of acid, and the stomach works harder to digest the larger amount of food.

- Avoid excessive grazing.
- Close the kitchen for business at least 2 or 3 hours before bedtime.
- Consider drinking in between meals instead of with meals to avoid excess stomach volume.

- Combine protein and fiber in each meal and consume four or five small meals and snacks throughout the day to help reduce or completely eliminate nighttime hunger.

If nighttime hunger persists, consider stocking up on low-sodium chicken broth or vegetable broth and sipping on it instead of eating solid food at night. Herbal teas may also help after dinner.

A Sample Day on the Acute Phase Diet

Let's take a look at what a sample day on the acute phase diet means for you:

Breakfast:

- $^1/_2$ cup dry oatmeal prepared with 1 cup fat-free milk plus 1 tablespoon brown sugar and $^1/_4$ teaspoon cinnamon for flavor
- 1 banana
- 1 cup herbal tea

Mid-morning snack:

- 1 cup fat-free Greek yogurt with $^1/_2$ banana and $^1/_4$ teaspoon vanilla extract mixed in for flavor

Lunch:

- 1 cup Ultimate Comfort Chicken Noodle Soup (recipe in Chapter 14)
- 1 Extraordinary Roast Beef Sandwich (recipe in Chapter 14)

Afternoon snack:

- 1 cup applesauce sprinkled with cinnamon plus 6 chopped walnuts

Dinner:

- 3 Baked Meatballs (recipe in Chapter 16) on top of mashed potatoes (skip the butter, pepper, and any fat-containing ingredients) plus 1 cup sautéed spinach (Consider using chicken broth instead of oil in the spinach to reduce the fat.)

TUMMY TAMER

Even though the restrictive elimination diet may alleviate your symptoms and make you feel good for a while, it's important to avoid any type of restrictive diet patterns long term to avoid potential nutrient deficiency.

The Chronic Symptom Control Diet

Once the acute symptoms pass, you may start reintroducing foods—one at a time, if possible—to determine your tolerance levels. Foods to try first include berries and other fruits, an extended selection of vegetables, and a wide array of allowed as well as questionable herbs and spices (see Chapter 8 for a list).

Caffeine is a well-known acid reflux trigger. If caffeine cravings overtake you or you *need* your java, consider trying a small cup of decaf and noting your symptoms. Alternatively, you could try espresso. Reports have shown it's better tolerated than the average large cup of coffee.

You may also consider trying various juices during this stage. Pear nectar and nectarine nectar may be better tolerated than citrus varieties. Overall, only reintroduce juices if absolutely necessary or in cases when weight gain may be your goal. Regardless of the acid reflux symptoms, liquid calories do not produce the same satiety as solid food, and eating solid fruits is a much better option for weight control.

Even though alcohol is not recommended and no amount has been shown to be definitively safe with acid reflux, you may consider trying small amounts of hard liquor or wine if absolutely necessary. Record your symptoms in your food journal. (You'll learn about food journals in the next section.)

ACID ALERT

Avoid consuming alcohol on an empty stomach, and never exceed the recommended intake of one drink per day for women and two drinks per day for men. One drink consists of 5 ounces wine, 12 ounces beer, or 1.5 ounces hard liquor.

Dear Diary: A Food Journal

Keeping a food journal is essential during the process of identifying trigger foods and those you tolerate well. I've included a sample food journal here; feel free to photocopy it and carry it with you. You also could record your food intake and symptoms in a separate notebook, or keep a detailed record in your computer or phone.

Food Journal

Date and Time	Food or Beverage	Portion Size	Symptoms

Be as specific as possible when filling out your food journal. Instead of recording simply "Green salad" in the Food or Beverage column, note what was in that green salad: "Raw spinach, raw cucumbers, canned beans, and olive oil." In the Portion Size column, list the amounts of each ingredient.

This method of record-keeping enables you to identify particular trigger foods and specific amounts that may provoke your acid reflux symptoms. For instance, you may be okay with 1 teaspoon olive oil but have a hard time eating $\frac{1}{4}$ cup poured over pasta or another dish.

Portion sizes are best recorded in tablespoons, teaspoons, cups, and other such specific measures. Recording "Large plate" is rather vague because the size of the plate is often in the eyes of the beholder. Furthermore, the plates can be overloaded with food or barely full.

The best way to determine portion sizes is to use your measuring spoons and cups. Consider measuring the foods you eat the most at least once to give you a good approximation of what a portion size looks like. Alternatively, you may use common household objects to approximate sizes:

- 1 CD case = 1 slice of bread
- 1 cup food is about the size of your fist.
- 1 (6-ounce) potato is about the size of a computer mouse.
- 3 or 4 ounces of meat is about the size of a deck of cards or your palm.

When filling out the Symptoms column, use a scale of 0 to 10, with 0 being the best you've ever felt and 10 being the worst reflux symptoms you've experienced.

In addition, in the Symptoms column, jot down notes if you experience gas, diarrhea, or other gastrointestinal distress after eating. Also note any questions you may want to address with your dietitian or physician or to research on your own later on.

It's almost like being your own detective. Ideally, you should be as specific as possible in your journal. Instead of saying "turkey sandwich," it's better to say "2 slices rye bread, 2 ounces roasted low-sodium turkey, 1 thin slice avocado, 1 teaspoon mayo, 2 small black olives." That way, you can start identifying whether it's the rye bread or another ingredient that's triggering your reflux when you compare one meal to the next.

TUMMY TAMER

If you make an appointment with a physician or a dietitian, be sure to bring along your food journal. It often holds the key to identifying your triggers and developing the best diet for you.

A Sample Day on the Chronic Phase Diet

Here's what a sample day on the chronic phase diet consists of:

Breakfast:

- 1 Airy Berry Pancake (recipe in Chapter 12)
- 2 tablespoons maple syrup
- 1 cup fat-free Greek yogurt
- 1 cup fat-free milk

Mid-morning snack:

- 1 cup fat-free cottage cheese plus 1 cup fresh berries

Lunch:

- 1 cup butternut squash soup
- 1 Apple Chicken Wrap (recipe in Chapter 14)

Afternoon snack:

- 2 tablespoons hummus (select a nonspicy variety) plus ½ cup baby carrots

Dinner:

- 1 Salmon Burger (recipe in Chapter 16)
- 1 serving Oven-Baked Fries (recipe in Chapter 20) or ¼ microwaved potato
- 2 cups roasted vegetables
- 1 slice Angel Food Cake with Berries (recipe in Chapter 21)

Heading to the Grocery Store

To eat an acid reflux–friendly diet, you might need certain foods and ingredients. Having those ingredients on hand, stocked in the pantry, refrigerator, or freezer, makes preparing reflux-friendly dishes a snap!

But before you depart for your shopping adventure, it helps to create a shopping list you can follow. Sticking to your list helps you spend less money on impulse buys and less healthy foods.

Smart Shopping Tips

The best place to start your shopping trip is in the produce section. Load up on fruits you can tolerate and ample vegetables.

To save money, consider buying produce that's in season or visiting your local farmers' market instead. You can sometimes find deliciously fresh food at markets.

Frozen and canned goods can be just as good as fresh—and often better—but be sure to read the labels and select items without any added salt, seasonings, or spices. Canned and frozen goods often have sauce added, as in the case of creamed spinach. It's best to purchase plain fruits and veggies and control what goes into the dish in your own kitchen.

At the meat counter, choose poultry without skin; pork tenderloin; Canadian bacon; and lean cuts of meat such as top round, top loin steak, tenderloin, flank steak, extra-lean ground beef, lean porterhouse, and sirloin. If you enjoy veal, opt for a loin chop, veal cutlets, or leg of lamb.

At the seafood counter, variety is your friend. Diversify your diet by incorporating whitefish, salmon, scallops, lobsters, and the rest.

TUMMY TAMER

If contamination, mercury poisoning, or fishing practices are a concern, visit the Monterey Bay Aquarium website (montereybayaquarium.org/cr/cr_seafoodwatch/sfw_recommendations.aspx) and download a brochure that explains various fish choices for you.

Staying along the perimeter of the store, next comes the dairy department. Load up on plain fat-free yogurts, fat-free milk, and fat-free cheese. (Avoid sharp varieties such as cheddar.) Reduced-fat butter can help flavor your food with little added fat and calories.

Now for eggs and egg whites. Egg whites are great because they're loaded with protein, have very few calories, and contain no added fat. You can separate your own eggs, discarding the yolk, or purchase containers of egg whites. If you opt for the store-bought containers, avoid already flavored options because they may contain acid reflux–unfriendly ingredients.

The danger zone—the store's center aisles—is where you'll find foods you should limit as much as possible: chips, heavily processed dressings, and desserts without an expiration date. Sticking to your list is essential here.

Only shop in the aisles you know you need something from, and only grab the items on your list. Among baking ingredients, stock up on flours, baking soda, baking powder, and cornstarch. In the herbs and spices section, pick up those included on your safe list (see Chapter 8). Snack foods such as rice cakes, popcorn, and whole-wheat crackers can be a great part of an acid reflux diet, but opt for the least-processed varieties.

Read the ingredient list and make sure that it is rather short. If it runs very long and there are many names you don't understand, don't buy the item. Some experts recommend sticking to items that have five or fewer ingredients listed on the ingredient list.

TUMMY TAMER

Consider buying items in bulk—especially when on sale—and freezing for later. Bread, fish, meat, and many fruits and vegetables freeze very well. And you'll be less tempted to try something you shouldn't when you have acid reflux–friendly foods on hand.

An Acid Reflux–Friendly Shopping List

The following is an easy-to-use shopping list. You can take it with you to the store as is or use it as a guide and create your own version.

Fruits:

- ❑ Apples
- ❑ Bananas
- ❑ Berries
- ❑ Cantaloupe
- ❑ Honeydew
- ❑ Papaya
- ❑ Other fruits depending on your tolerance

Vegetables:

- ❑ Asparagus
- ❑ Beets
- ❑ Brussels sprouts
- ❑ Cabbage
- ❑ Carrots—shredded and baby
- ❑ Cauliflower
- ❑ Celery
- ❑ Corn
- ❑ Cucumbers
- ❑ Eggplant
- ❑ Kale
- ❑ Mushrooms
- ❑ Peas
- ❑ Potatoes
- ❑ Spinach
- ❑ Squash
- ❑ Sweet potatoes
- ❑ Zucchini

Whole grains:

- ❑ Amaranth
- ❑ Barley
- ❑ Brown rice
- ❑ Buckwheat
- ❑ Bulgur wheat
- ❑ Couscous (whole-wheat)
- ❑ Millet
- ❑ Oats
- ❑ Popcorn
- ❑ Quinoa

continues

continued

- ❑ Rye
- ❑ Spelt
- ❑ Whole-wheat pasta
- ❑ Wild rice

Canned goods:

- ❑ Blueberries without sugar
- ❑ No-salt-added beans
- ❑ 100 percent pumpkin purée
- ❑ Soup (Check that the ingredients are acid reflux friendly.)
- ❑ Unsweetened applesauce
- ❑ Vegetables without salt

Snacks:

- ❑ Baked potato chips
- ❑ Dried prunes
- ❑ Graham crackers
- ❑ Low-sodium pretzels
- ❑ Plain popcorn
- ❑ Rice cakes
- ❑ Whole-wheat crackers

Oils and dressings:

- ❑ Canola oil
- ❑ Light plant sterol and stanol spreads (Benecol)
- ❑ Natural almond butter
- ❑ Natural cashew butter
- ❑ Natural peanut butter
- ❑ Nonstick cooking spray
- ❑ Olive oil

- ❑ Peanut oil
- ❑ Sesame oil
- ❑ Truffle oil

Herbs and spices:

- ❑ Basil
- ❑ Chamomile
- ❑ Cilantro
- ❑ Cinnamon
- ❑ Coriander
- ❑ Dill
- ❑ Ginger
- ❑ Licorice
- ❑ Oregano
- ❑ Parsley
- ❑ Rosemary
- ❑ Sugar (granulated, brown, confectioners')
- ❑ Tarragon
- ❑ Thyme
- ❑ Turmeric
- ❑ Vanilla extract

Dairy:

- ❑ Fat-free cottage cheese
- ❑ Fat-free milk
- ❑ Fat-free mozzarella cheese
- ❑ Fat-free or low-fat ricotta cheese
- ❑ Fat-free sour cream
- ❑ Fat-free yogurt, Greek
- ❑ Fat-free yogurt, plain
- ❑ Low-fat kefir

continues

continued

- ❑ Reduced-fat feta cheese
- ❑ Reduced-fat provolone cheese
- ❑ Reduced-fat shredded Parmesan cheese
- ❑ Reduced-fat Swiss cheese

Eggs:

- ❑ Eggs
- ❑ Flavor-free egg whites
- ❑ Hard-boiled and peeled eggs

Meat:

- ❑ Lean cuts of lamb
- ❑ Lean cuts of pork
- ❑ Lean cuts of veal
- ❑ Lean ground beef
- ❑ Lean ground turkey
- ❑ Lean poultry

Fish:

- ❑ Albacore tuna
- ❑ Bluefish
- ❑ Cod
- ❑ Eel
- ❑ Flounder
- ❑ Haddock
- ❑ Halibut
- ❑ Herring
- ❑ Mackerel
- ❑ Red snapper
- ❑ Sea bass

Seafood:

- ❑ Crab
- ❑ Crayfish
- ❑ Lobster
- ❑ Scallops
- ❑ Shrimp

Frozen foods:

- ❑ Fat-free vanilla ice cream
- ❑ Frozen berries
- ❑ Frozen fish
- ❑ Frozen papaya chunks
- ❑ Frozen vegetables without sauce or spices

The Least You Need to Know

- When you experience severe pain and acute acid reflux symptoms, avoid all known and questionable trigger foods.
- For chronic reflux management, keep a detailed food journal and identify your personal triggers while incorporating more foods back into your diet.
- A few small, structured meals are better than one large one.
- Stop eating at least 2 or 3 hours before bedtime to avoid triggering your reflux symptoms.

Making Sense of Exercise

Chapter 7

In This Chapter

- The connection between exercise and acid reflux
- Acid reflux–friendly activities
- Fun ways to burn calories
- Getting the food fuel you need
- The importance of hydration

Exercise helps you manage your weight, live a pain-free life, improve your cardiovascular health, slow down aging, prevent chronic diseases, and help your heart beat longer. Exercise comes in many forms, but if you have acid reflux, you need to choose your activities carefully because the wrong exercise could cause your acid reflux to flare up. For instance, running, when done right, helps reduce reflux symptoms. And that's just one option. I describe a plethora of other activities that help you do the same in this chapter.

It's important to note that no movement happens without proper nutrition and hydration. Knowledge about the acid reflux–friendly ways to fuel your body is the key to reducing your symptoms while increasing your performance. This chapter not only helps you understand the ins and outs of sports nutrition, but also provides helpful tips on how to implement them into your daily life. You'll be the talk of the locker room in no time!

The Benefits of Physical Activity

It's a no-brainer that exercise should be an essential part of your life. Staying active with acid reflux can be tricky, but it's far from impossible. Although your uncomfortable reflux symptoms might make you want to avoid exercising, know this: exercise not only can be a great way to pass time, it can actually help alleviate some of your reflux symptoms, too.

Physical activity has a positive effect on *gastric motility*, or the movement of food through your digestive tract. Moving your body helps sustain the stomach muscle contractions, called *peristalsis*, that facilitate timely stomach emptying. This is particularly important because slow gastric emptying is one of the causes of reflux. To avoid unwanted and potentially harmful by-products of food staying in your digestive tract, exercise helps move things along by stimulating the intestines.

DEFINITION

Gastric motility refers to the movement of the stomach that helps direct contents from the stomach to the small intestines. **Peristalsis** is a medical term that describes the smooth, rhythmic, wavelike contractions of the intestines or other tubular structure that propel contents through the digestive tract.

The most important benefit exercise can have on your body in relation to acid reflux is weight management. Excess weight creates additional pressure around your midsection, squeezing your stomach and creating unwanted pressure for your LES. Shedding the pounds helps you shed that unwanted abdominal pressure. Being able to flaunt your toned midsection is an added bonus!

Finding the Right Acid Reflux–Friendly Exercises

You can enjoy and benefit from a plethora of exercises without having a flare-up. The main idea when selecting exercises is to focus not only on the type of activity, but on the intensity, body positioning, and duration because those factors are critical to keep acid reflux at bay.

Rate of Perceived Exertion

High-intensity activities have been known to exacerbate acid reflux symptoms, so staying within a light- to moderate-intensity level of exercise is key. The rate of perceived exertion (RPE) is a great way to measure intensity during training to help you be sure your exercise remains acid reflux free.

RPE is measured on a 0 to 10 scale. Zero is considered the least intense, equal to watching TV or sleeping. Ten is equivalent to the highest intensity, comparable to running away from a bear.

Rate of Perceived Exertion (RPE)

0	Nothing at all
1	Very weak
2	Weak
3	Weak/moderate
4	Moderate
5	Moderate/strong
6	Strong
7	Very strong
8	Very, very strong
9	Extremely strong
10	The highest level of intensity (The body is only capable of short, less than a minute, intense bouts of such exercise.)

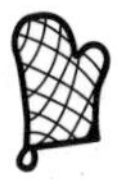

COOLER TALK

The RPE scale was originally developed by Gunnar Borg in 1982. Called the Borg Scale, it ranged from 6 to 20. In 1986, the American College of Sports Medicine modified it to the present 0 to 10 scale. Some fitness professionals still prefer to use the Borg Scale.

At the beginning of any exercise program, it's best to start with easier movements and gradually increase the intensity of your workouts so you can better gauge your response to exercise. Try to stay within the 4 to 5 range, which yields optimal health benefits without worsening acid reflux symptoms. Some people may only tolerate level 3 for the first week but then are able to increase. If you feel symptoms after the start of exercise, immediately decrease the intensity of your movements until your symptoms subside.

What's My Heart Rate?

Heart rate is another fantastic tool you can use to measure your level of exercise intensity. Knowing this number can help you gauge your progress as well as steer clear of reflux. The American Heart Association recommends exercising at the target heart rate range of 50 to 85 percent of your maximum heart rate. However, those with acid reflux should not exceed 70 percent of their maximal heart rate. So what does this mean for you?

Your target heart rate tells you the appropriate number of heart beats per minute where you can reap the most cardiovascular benefits while still staying safe. The formula and the calculations are rather basic:

$$220 - \text{age} = X$$

Multiply X by the multiplier, which in this case is 50 percent for the lower limit and 70 percent for the upper limit. For example, Bob, a 30-year-old with acid reflux, wants to figure an appropriate heart rate range prior to beginning his workout routine. Here's how he'd do it:

$$220 - 30 = 190$$

$$190 \times 50\% \text{ (or 0.5)} = 95 \text{ beats per minute}$$

$$190 \times 70\% \text{ (or 0.70)} = 133 \text{ beats per minute}$$

Bob's range is 95 to 133 beats per minute.

TUMMY TAMER

The target heart rate for the acid reflux population (50 to 70 percent max heart rate) corresponds to 4 to 5 on the RPE scale. If you have a hard time calculating your heart rate, you can safely use the RPE scale instead.

Proper Body Positioning

Did you ever have a snack followed by some intense crunches at the gym? If so, the pain you experienced after exercising probably taught you that not all exercises are created equal when it comes to acid reflux. You can—and should—stay active when working with gastric reflux. However, knowing what type of moves and body positions may trigger your reflux enables you to modify your routine while still enjoying your favorite activities.

Your body should always be in the upright position. Sports and activities that require getting horizontal, or in a supine position, are not acid reflux friendly. Excessive shaking and up-and-down motions can also trigger unwanted symptoms. Examples of activities to avoid include surfing, abdominal work on the floor, some yoga and Pilates positions, acrobatics, diving, and excessive bending in the abdominal region.

More Is Not Always Better

As a general rule for those living with acid reflux, the lower the intensity, the longer you can perform the activity without aggravating your acid reflux. That means ultra-endurance events such as marathons, especially Ironman triathlons, are not advised. Exercising for an hour at proper intensity and proper body positioning probably won't trigger your acid reflux symptoms. Exercise that goes beyond an hour, however, may cause a flare-up.

To avoid symptoms, increase your activity gradually. A good rule of thumb is to increase the progress of your exercise routine by 10 minutes every week.

Acid Reflux–Friendly Exercises

Now that you know all about how to properly move, let's look at a list of acid reflux–friendly exercises. Always remember that exercise comes in many forms and sizes, with gym routines making up only a small portion of the active lifestyle you can lead.

Acid Reflux–Friendly Exercises*

Activity	Calories Burned per Hour
Aerobics, low impact	375
Boating	150
Bowling	165

continues

Acid Reflux-Friendly Exercises* (continued)

Activity	Calories Burned per Hour
Boxing, moderate intensity	350
Calisthenics, light	200
Canoeing, light/moderate	185
Cycling, light/moderate	350
Dance (salsa, tap, ballroom), light	255
Frisbee playing	170
Gardening	235
Golfing (without the golf cart)	255
Hiking with backpack	400
Ice skating, moderate	400
Running, light (5 miles per hour)	465
Ski machine, moderate	400
Skiing (downhill or water), moderate	350
Snow shoeing	465
Tai Chi	235
Walking	200
Water aerobics (upright)	350
Weight lifting, light/moderate	175
Yoga (some moves may aggravate reflux)	235

**Calorie estimates are based on a 150-pound person.*

Now that you know what exercises are good to try if acid reflux bothers you, let's look at some exercises you should avoid. In general, don't carry heavy objects. When it comes to exercise, avoid basketball, football, gymnastics, martial arts, intense running and sprinting, snowboarding, soccer, surfing, swimming and diving, tennis, and wrestling. In the gym, avoid *plyometrics*, intense weight lifting, powerlifting, deadlifting, and flat bench pressing.

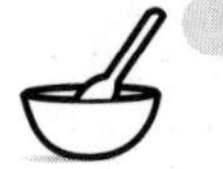

DEFINITION

Plyometrics is a type of physical training style designed to produce explosive, rapid, and powerful movements for the purpose of improving sports performance. It is not advised for acid reflux sufferers.

Weight Lifting Substitutions

You likely noticed weightlifting on the no-no list. Just because you have acid reflux, that doesn't mean you should discontinue your resistance-training routine. The following table offers some suggestions of acid reflux–friendly options to replace traditional exercises.

Instead of This ...	Try This ...
Flat bench barbell press	Seated machine chest press
Leg press	Machine squat
Bent-over row	Seated machine row
Crunches on the floor	Hanging knee raises
Flat bench dumbbell press	Seated machine chest fly
Dumbbell row	Cable lat pull-down

All fitness facilities carry different types of equipment, so look for machines that exercise your body in the upright position. Steer clear of machines and exercises that put your body in the supine position or make you bend at the torso.

Physical Activity Guidelines

Now that you've been persuaded exercise is good for you, how much do you actually need? According to the Centers for Disease Control and Prevention, for optimal health, adults should exercise for 150 minutes per week at moderate intensity levels of aerobic activity. In addition, two or more resistance-training workouts are advised. The recommendation is to execute at least one set per muscle group for 8 to 12 repetitions.

Creativity and enjoyment are important for adhering to any type of routine. If you select acid reflux–friendly exercises, you're also less likely to experience the postexercise burn, which will help you stick with your routine.

Getting Help Getting Moving

If this is the first time you're setting out on an exercise routine and you are intimidated by the look of the dumbbells and the other confusing-looking equipment in the gym, don't be. Many qualified professionals can teach you how to use the machines, use the correct form, develop a fun and diverse exercise routine, and ensure you're getting a great workout while steering clear of the acid reflux–provoking movements.

Trainers, like many other professionals, come in a variety of shapes and sizes. To find the best and most qualified match for you, look for his or her credentials.

ACSM (American College of Sports Medicine) requires a current CPR certification and an undergraduate degree in exercise physiology or any related field.

ACE (American College on Exercise) requires a current CPR certification and is a nationally approved organization. The downside to ACE is the program design is not as integrated as NASM and ACSM. Note that this is not a reflection on a trainer's ability to develop a successful routine.

NASM (National Academy of Sports Medicine) requires a current CPR certification. NASM is known for its signature five-phase program design, which is backed by science and is used by many fitness professionals.

Once you've identified the right trainer for you, don't be afraid to interview the person. Here are some questions to consider asking:

- Is your certification current? What kind of continuing education are you involved in?
- How many months/years of experience do you have?
- Can I get references from your existing or prior clients?
- How often do you work with people who have reflux, and how would you go about developing a program for this condition?
- If I purchase a package of sessions, will they ever expire?
- Is there a cancellation fee if I need to cancel an appointment?
- Would you be willing to write out my program and give me homework I can follow between our sessions?

An experienced and qualified trainer should be able to answer all these questions. If he or she doesn't, continue looking. Many trainers may even offer a complimentary workout to get you started to see if you are a good match for each other.

Fueling with Acid Reflux

Proper nourishment is essential for a good exercise session. After all, who can spend an hour at the gym in a hungry state and expect his or her body to work out at peak performance without sufficient nutrients? For acid reflux sufferers, this issue presents a particular challenge.

Timing Is Everything

Eating too close to your workout and hydrating with common beverages such as flavored drinks and protein shakes may exacerbate your symptoms. If you were hoping to use this as an excuse to avoid exercise, not so fast! You can eat, drink, and still find success at the gym.

First, adjust your meal timing around your workouts. Don't eat anything or drink anything other than water for at least an hour, or even two hours, prior to exercising.

Many people use exercise as an excuse to eat more. But unless you're a marathon runner or participate in other ultra-endurance sports, you should be able to handle an hour or two of exercise eating the same number of calories you normally eat. You could have a snack one hour before exercise and your dinner when you get home. Or you could split your dinner in two and have one half one hour before and the other half upon completion of the exercise routine. Or have one snack an hour before and one snack as soon as you're done. This is especially pertinent to those who tend to experience episodes of *hypoglycemia* during exercise and may need to replenish as soon as they hit the locker room.

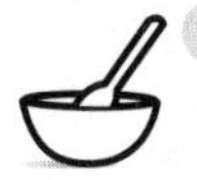

DEFINITION

Hypoglycemia is a condition in which a person has an abnormally low level of blood sugar. It can result from prolonged exercise, poor diet, and excessive insulin production.

Food as Fuel

Now let's look at what you should eat and what should be the breakdown of macronutrients before and after your workout. It's a good idea to fuel up primarily on carbohydrates, with small amounts of protein and some fat.

Just as the timing of your pre-exercise meal is important for reflux management, the timing of your postexercise meal is imperative for proper muscle repair and restoration of the glycogen stores for your next session. It's recommended that you replenish your body by consuming a meal rich in protein and carbohydrates within 4 hours after completing exercise. However, it's even better to consume a meal within an hour after the end of exercise because this is when your "metabolic" window is open the widest. In other words, the absorption of nutrients is maximized during the first hour following the exercise.

The recommended dietary intake of carbohydrates for an active adult is 2 to 10 grams per kilogram of body weight per day. If you're a moderately active person, stay closer to the 2-gram mark. If you're closer to an ultra-endurance athlete, stick to the higher end of the recommended range.

The recommended protein intake for a moderately active person is 0.8 grams/kg/day. If you strength-train or participate in endurance events, however, increase your consumption to 1.2 to 1.7 grams/kg/day. For your postworkout meal, choose natural sources of protein over protein powders because natural foods contain a perfect blend of amino acids, are more filling, and do not contain unnecessary chemicals and additives frequently added to protein powders.

It's advised to consume 30 grams carbohydrates 1 or 2 hours before exercise and 25 to 50 grams protein and 30 to 60 grams carbohydrates after exercise.

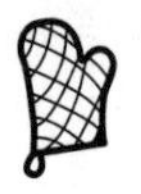

COOLER TALK

Did you know: 1 kilogram is 2.2 pounds? Therefore, a 150-pound person weighs 68.2 kilograms (150 ÷ 2.2). The proper protein consumption for that person is between 82 grams (68.2 × 1.2) and 116 grams (68.2 × 1.7) per day.

Smart Snacking

Now that you understand the macronutrient breakdown, let's translate it into real food. The following are great choices for preworkout snacks:

- 1 banana and 10 almonds
- 2 figs with 1 ounce low-fat string cheese
- Low-fat yogurt and 1 small banana

- Smoothie (1 banana, 1 cup fat-free milk or soy milk, a few ice cubes, ¼ teaspoon vanilla extract, 1 teaspoon ground flaxseed)
- Yogurt parfait (low-fat yogurt with ¼ cup granola)
- 6 whole-wheat crackers plus ½ tablespoon peanut butter
- 1 diced pear sprinkled with 1 tablespoon flaxseed and 1 tablespoon honey
- ¾ cup fat-free cottage cheese with ½ cup cubed melon, drizzled with 1 tablespoon honey

Amazingly delicious postworkout treats may consist of the following:

- Smoothie (1 banana, 1 cup fat-free milk or soy milk, 1 cup fat-free plain yogurt, a few ice cubes, ¼ teaspoon vanilla extract, 1 teaspoon ground flaxseed)
- 1 cup vanilla fat-free yogurt topped with ½ cubed melon
- 3 ounces low-fat string cheese slices with 1 golden delicious apple
- 3 ounces toasted soybean nuts
- 1 cup low-fat plain yogurt mixed with ½ cup granola

If you're working out close to dinnertime and you're comfortable waiting to get your postworkout nutrition at dinner, you can forgo your snack and have a meal. Be sure you're not ravenous when the dinner is served, though, because that can lead you to overeat.

The Importance of Hydration

Proper hydration is vital during prolonged exercise. If you're like many reflux sufferers, you've probably noticed that many flavored *electrolyte* drinks, carbonated beverages, and protein shakes have exacerbated your symptoms. So what are you to do?

DEFINITION

Electrolytes are substances that give the body capacity to conduct electricity, an essential function for our cells and organs. Typical electrolyte solutions contain sodium, potassium, and chloride.

First, start by conducting a "sweat test" to assess how much liquid you lose during exercise. Weigh yourself before and after you work out. Subtract your weight after from your weight before, add the amount of water you consumed during your workout, and you'll get the net liquid lost.

Let's say, for example, that after conducting a sweat test, you calculated that you lost 32 ounces of fluid during your workout. Eight ounces = 1 cup, so you should consume at least 4 cups fluids during your workouts to maintain the proper hydration.

Water has been shown to be the best fluid for hydration. If the sight and smell of plain water doesn't do it for you, consider making a homemade herbal tea, cooling it in the refrigerator, and bringing it with you. Or flavor your water by adding a little ginger and 1 teaspoon honey for sweetness.

The average person moving his or her body for a couple hours—even during periods of heavy exertion—does not require special rehydration solutions like those bottled electrolyte drinks. However, if you want to boost your electrolytes, here's a recipe for a homemade electrolyte solution that won't exacerbate your acid reflux symptoms. (This is also a great way to hydrate during periods of food-borne illnesses such as vomiting and diarrhea.)

Homemade Electrolyte Solution

1 l water

8 tsp. sugar

1 tsp. table salt

1/4 tsp. baking soda

1/2 cup mashed banana for flavor (optional)

Simply combine all the ingredients in a water bottle, and you're good to go. You even can make this solution ahead of time and store it in the refrigerator. It's acid reflux friendly, inexpensive, and doesn't contain any artificial coloring or preservatives like sports drinks often do.

Now that you're equipped with all this information about nutrition and exercise, it's time to get active. Start today, and don't wait until tomorrow! Your body will thank you for it.

The Least You Need to Know

- Select exercises that will keep you in the upright position and avoid excessive bouncing.
- Opt for activities you enjoy most so you can more easily meet the recommended 150 minutes of physical activity per week.
- When in doubt at the gym, let a qualified trainer help you.
- Avoid eating for 1 or 2 hours before exercising.
- Stay hydrated with water and don't use your exercise routine as an excuse to eat more food!

Part 3

Cooking and Dining Out Strategies

Starting a new diet or way of eating can be intimidating, but it needn't be. In Part 3, I share some tips to help you feel more comfortable in the kitchen while you're preparing acid reflux–friendly foods. I also give you shopping lists for what foods to buy and especially what to avoid.

Holidays, dining out, and traveling are all fun parts of life. But the temptations and traditional dishes accompanying each occasion may make it difficult to adhere to an acid reflux diet. This part provides you with specific menu ideas you can order when eating out, plus other tools you need to make navigating these situations a cinch.

In the Kitchen

Chapter 8

In This Chapter

- Acid reflux–friendly spices and herbs
- The best cooking techniques for acid reflux
- More flavor with less reflux
- Ingredient substitutions and flavor combinations

Having control over what you eat is one of the biggest steps toward an acid reflux–free life. Even if you don't consider yourself a good cook, don't be discouraged! This chapter provides all the tools you need to cook healthy, tasty, and make-you-feel-good dishes and snacks.

In the culinary world, fat is the main precursor for flavor. But for reflux sufferers, excess fat consumption isn't recommended, especially in the form of flavorings. It not only aggravates your symptoms; it also adds extra calories to your daily calorie allotment. This is where herbs and spices come to the rescue. Knowing how to flavor your food not only keeps your palate satisfied, it also elevates your nutrition because many herbs and spices are great sources of vitamins, minerals, antioxidants, phytonutrients, and other beneficial compounds. And they're all virtually calorie free!

Once you learn how to flavor your food, it's important to use proper reflux-approved cooking techniques that can help you achieve perfect-tasting dishes. Finally, the useful tips in this chapter can help you save money and be more proficient in the kitchen. So let's get started!

Herbs and Spices

Even though substantial research has been conducted identifying trigger herbs and spices, the final list will be individual because degree of tolerance varies from person to person. In general, anything that's "hot," "spicy," or "acidic" should not be part of your diet. The following table outlines other herbs and spices. Some you need to steer clear of to avoid flare-ups, some are safe to enjoy, and some are worth experimenting with.

The Good	Worth Experimenting With	Better to Avoid
Basil	Cardamom	Black pepper
Chamomile	Garlic powder	Cayenne
Cilantro	Onion powder	Chile peppers
Cinnamon	Paprika	Cloves
Coriander	Saffron	Curry
Dill	Salt	Habañero
Ginger	Star anise	Jalapeño
Licorice		Mint
Oregano		Mustard
Parsley		Nutmeg
Rosemary		Peppermint
Sugar		
Tarragon		
Thyme		
Turmeric		
Vanilla		

Generally, powders are better tolerated than whole seeds or those that are coarsely ground. So if you really enjoy certain herbs that are on the "avoid" list, try them in powdered form and introduce gradually, closely monitoring how you feel. Herbs and spices that are on the acceptable list should be consumed in fresh form whenever possible.

Tasty Flavor Combinations

Knowing what to eat is the first part. It's also important to know how to use those ingredients to create a delicious experience. In this section, I give you a guide to help you understand how to puzzle all the flavor pieces together. Feel free to ignite your creative spark and go beyond these suggestions to create your own flavorful combinations.

Basil, with its warm, slightly peppery yet dominant flavor, is perfect for stuffing poultry and flavoring soups and gravies. Traditionally, basil goes well with garlic and tomatoes, but for those with acid reflux, that combination would be off the list.

Chamomile, aside from making stomach-soothing tea, is delicious paired with honey, figs, and ice cream.

Cilantro is a perfect finish to a dish. Use fresh cilantro to garnish meat, poultry, fish, pasta, and virtually any main course.

Cinnamon, one of the oldest spices known to man, is great to soothe the stomach—an ideal natural acid reflux remedy. Add cinnamon to apple pie, pudding, rice, Greek yogurt, ice cream, beef, or lamb stew. Cooked fruit is perfect for those with acid reflux, and by adding cinnamon, you'll elevate the flavor even more.

Fresh *coriander*, similar to cilantro, pairs well with meats, sauces, stir-fry, soups, and salads.

Dill has a clean and grassy taste and a variety of uses. Famous applications include cucumber dill dressing, potato salad, garnish for salmon and other types of fish, cream cheese, and herb butter.

ACID ALERT

To avoid reflux flare-ups, stay away from dill pickles. They're acidic due to their high vinegar content.

Ginger does wonders to alleviate acid reflux symptoms. It pairs well with chicken, beef, and tea. Ginger is often used to flavor curry dishes and goes well with curry powder, which may trigger acid reflux. Be sure to stay away from this flavor combination.

Licorice, a bittersweet root, can be used to flavor barley, gingerbread, teas, and syrups—in addition to its use in making candy.

Oregano's earthy flavor and minty aroma go well with vegetables and bean dishes. Sprinkle dried oregano on your salad, scrambled eggs, or sautéed zucchini.

Parsley has a light scent and fresh taste and is acid reflux friendly. Add parsley to tabbouleh, garnish your meat or poultry dish with it for additional flavor and a finished look, or pair it with rice dishes and chickpea salads.

Rosemary's aroma and long-lasting flavor make it ideal for cooking. The best use of rosemary is with potatoes and lamb. You can also sprinkle it over ice cream or mousse, cook it in with vegetables, or use it in chicken or beef marinades.

Salt is a common item in most kitchens. Even though salt is a useful flavor-enhancing agent, studies have shown that high salt consumption leads to the exacerbation of acid reflux. If you stick to the recommended daily allowance equivalent of 1 teaspoon, you should be in the green.

Sugar is another popular kitchen staple. Sugar adds sweetness to dishes but also empty calories, so use it in moderation. Substituting sugar with honey is worth experimenting with. Avoid substituting sugar with artificial sweeteners because those have been shown to worsen acid reflux.

Tarragon, with its strong flavor, is best used to infuse oil. With the increased flavor, you're more likely to use less oil to satisfy your palate, which not only should help keep your reflux symptoms in check but also should keep down the fat in your diet.

Add slightly pungent *thyme* to breads, potatoes, mushrooms, vegetables, and omelets.

Turmeric's flavor creates a perfect *mouthfeel*. Best paired with beans, potatoes, cauliflower, or lentils, turmeric is also added to high-fat foods like butters and sauces, so avoid those types of foods if at all possible.

DEFINITION

Mouthfeel refers to the overall sensation in the mouth resulting from a combination of temperature, taste, smell, and texture of food.

Vanilla is one of the most popular flavorings in the kitchen. If you're a chocolate lover, vanilla serves as a great substitute to alleviate sweet-tooth cravings. In general, vanilla enhances the flavor of a dish. Add it to baked goods, but also pair it with fresh fruit, teas, and ice cream.

One of the great benefits of herbs and spices is their long shelf life. However, when you buy fresh herbs, use them as quickly as possible to preserve their freshness and reap the maximum nutrients.

Smart Substitutions

Old habits are hard to break, especially when it comes to food. However, living with acid reflux is unpleasant, to say the least, and can lead to much more serious health conditions. So to help you make a smooth transition to an acid reflux–friendly diet—without compromising your old favorites—I share the information in the following table.

As with spices, a good rule of thumb is to avoid anything with extreme flavor, but if there's something you can't resist, slow introduction is a must. Choose lower-fat options, and you'll come out a winner.

ACID ALERT

Be sure, when swapping ingredients, that no high-fructose corn syrup or artificial sweeteners are included in the ingredients list. They may make your acid reflux worse.

Instead of This ...	Try This ...
Bacon (traditional)	Canadian bacon.
Beef burger	Veggie burger, chickpea burger, portobello mushroom burger, lean turkey burger, ostrich burger, or bison burger.
Beef pot pie	Canned stew (or homemade low-sodium stew is even better!) with a crust made from reduced-fat biscuit mix.
Butter or margarine	Low-fat margarine, light butter (may need to add more flour when baking), or apple butter.
Cheddar cheese	2 percent cheddar cheese.
Chocolate pie	Vanilla pudding made with skim milk and crushed graham crackers as crust.
Chocolate-chip cookie	Vanilla or chocolate rice cakes, vanilla wafers, ginger-snaps, fig bars, or animal crackers.
Coffee creamer	Fat-free creamer or half-and-half.
Cream cheese	Fat-free cream cheese, tofu cream cheese (dairy free).

continues

continued

Instead of This …	Try This …
Cream-based soup	Broth-based soup, miso soup.
Creamy dressings	Fat-free Greek yogurt cucumber dill dip.
Egg, 1 large	2 egg whites.
Egg roll	Steamed pork dumplings.
Fish sticks	Homemade sticks prepared with whole-wheat breadcrumbs; sprinkle with vegetable oil and bake instead of frying. For the dipping sauce, use Tzatziki Yogurt Dip (recipe in Chapter 13).
Fruit juice	Fresh, nonacidic fruit juice or whole fresh fruit; dilute your juice with water (70 percent juice, 30 percent water), and add ice to help decrease reflux symptoms.
Gravy	Beef, chicken, or vegetable broth thickened with cornstarch or *agar agar*.
Ground beef	95 to 99 percent lean ground beef, veal.
Heavy cream	Evaporated skim milk.
Hot fudge topping	Vanilla topping.
Ice cream	Low-fat frozen yogurt, sorbet, sherbet, or gelato in a less-acidic flavor such as vanilla or banana as opposed to orange or lemon.
Maple syrup	Light maple syrup.
Mayonnaise	Nonfat or "lite" canola mayonnaise.
Oil used during baking	Unsweetened applesauce, apple butter, pear butter, puréed prunes, or avocado.
Onion rings	Steamed vegetables, baked kale chips with sea salt.
Pastrami, salami	Lean roast beef or lean turkey.
Pork loin	Pork tenderloin.
Pork sausage	Extra-lean turkey sausage.
Porterhouse steak or chuck	Tenderloin, top round, lamb shank, or ostrich steak.
Pound cake with berries	Angel food cake with a banana.
Ricotta cheese	Fat-free ricotta cheese or firm tofu.
Shortening (for baking)	Ratio of 1/2 nonfat cream cheese and 1/2 margarine.
Soda, soft drinks	Iced herbal tea.
Sour cream	Fat-free Greek yogurt.
Tuna in oil (canned)	Tuna in water or low-sodium vegetable broth.
Whipped cream	Whipped evaporated milk.
Whole milk	Buttermilk.

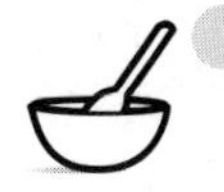

DEFINITION

Agar agar is a gelling agent traditionally used in Asian cuisine for making desserts. Agar is derived from red algae. Its gelling capability and bland flavor make it versatile for making not only desserts but also soups, sauces, and gravies.

Reflux-Friendly Cooking Techniques

Acid reflux should not preclude you from having fun in the kitchen. Many different cooking techniques can be used to add flavor and diversify the texture of your dishes. Just imagine how different a fillet of salmon can taste if it is grilled, broiled, or poached. Using the right cooking method can also add juiciness to a lean cut of meat or crispiness to a fish fillet.

If you don't have a grill, an inexpensive stovetop grill can add great flavor year-round.

Baking is a method of heat transfer through hot air. The food is surrounded by hot air from all sides. Baking is efficient because large quantities of food can be prepared at one time, and it's a very low-maintenance cooking method. It's also one of the healthiest ways to prepare your food, whether you suffer from acid reflux or not.

Braising combines dry and moist heat cooking methods. Typically, meat is an ideal food to braise. First, the meat is pan sautéed on high heat until it's light brown on each side. The heat is then reduced, liquid is added, and the dish is cooked at low temperature until ready. This method results in a rich flavor. Just like with stewing, leaner cuts of meat are typically used with this method. It's ideal for those with acid reflux.

Broiling is a cooking method wherein heat radiates onto the food from the top. This method is wonderful because it uses high heat and enables you to achieve browning on the finished product, which adds flavor without additional calories. This method is useful in combination with baking or other cooking methods as well. Use it as a finishing touch to your dish—there's nothing more satisfying than a sizzle!

Grilling is a dry cooking method in which the heat is radiated from the bottom. This method is efficient because you can cook your protein, starches, and fruit all at the same time. Grilling helps reduce the fat content of meat because the fat drips down and away from the meat as it melts and liquefies. Plus, the smoky flavor it imparts to the food will have you coming back for more.

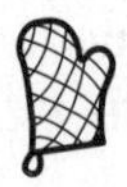

COOLER TALK

Grilling is one of the oldest cooking techniques known to man, dating as far back as 1.4 million years. Our ancestors realized grilling adds a lot of flavor without the use of additional flavorings, even if they didn't realize then how beneficial this would be to future acid reflux sufferers!

Poaching is a moist heat cooking method wherein food is submerged in a liquid and cooked at a range of 165°F to 168°F. Commonly poached foods include eggs, fruit, poultry, and fish. The two main reflux-friendly benefits of poaching are the transfer of flavor and the acid reduction of some foods. For instance, fish or chicken can be poached in a vegetable stock that allows for enhanced flavor and tender texture. When fruit is cooked using this method, it loses its acidity, which you'll love if you have acid reflux. So if you absolutely crave citrus fruit such as grapefruit or oranges, this may be your best option, but again, tread carefully.

Pressure cooking, unlike other moist cooking methods, uses the least amount of liquid because the minimal amount used is evaporated during the cooking process. Pressure cooking produces similar results to boiling, poaching, or stewing but is much quicker. Additionally, because of the "closed system" design, few vitamins and minerals escape, making pressure cooking one of the preferred methods of food preparation.

Anytime you submerge food into water for cooking, some of the water-soluble vitamins leach out. That's why when you boil broccoli, the water turns green. *Steaming* does not have the same leaching problem because your food is held above the water and is being cooked by hot steam, not in the hot water. It's a perfect solution for those with acid reflux because steaming maximizes the retention of essential vitamins and minerals in your food.

Stewing is a slow, moist cooking method that uses much less water than boiling. It's typically used to cook leaner cuts of meat because they require a longer cooking time to achieve desired tenderness. Prolonged cooking allows the excess liquid to evaporate, concentrating the flavors of the dish.

Cooking Techniques to Avoid

Now that we've covered the good techniques for you to use when cooking an acid reflux–friendly diet, let's look at those to avoid.

Pan-frying, deep-frying, sautéing, and stir-frying using a lot of oil are all cooking methods that will aggravate acid reflux symptoms.

Another common pitfall is the use of high-fat marinades during meat, poultry, and fish preparation. Choose lower-fat options, or use herbs and spices to exclude fat altogether.

Cooking Tips

I've given you a lot of information already, but before I turn you loose to start digging in to the recipes and cooking acid reflux–friendly dishes, here are some of the cooking tips that are regularly practiced in my family. I hope some can make it into your kitchen as well!

Use a paper towel slightly damp with oil to wipe a skillet or saucepan instead of pouring oil into it. You'll use far less oil for cooking.

Purchase a manual oil spray pump. It saves you money in the long run and gives you control over what kind of and how much oil you use for your dishes. Spraying oil as opposed to pouring it provides the right amount of flavor with built-in portion control.

Invest in a cast-iron pan and grill top. If you follow the manufacturer's care instructions, cast iron will last you a lifetime. With time and proper seasoning, these pans add flavor and additional iron to your meals. Invest in a cast-iron grill pan, and you'll enjoy grilling indoors year 'round!

Purchase an 8-inch chef's knife. It's versatile enough to be used for fine chopping and even butchering larger cuts of meat.

Invest in a hand blender so you can blend fruit and vegetables into soups, purées, and desserts without bulky cooking equipment.

Purchase good measuring cups and spoons. Opt for stainless-steel cups and spoons with imprinted measurements because paint fades away with time.

It's worth investing in glass storage containers because glass is a safer material in which to store food. Plus, glass lasts considerably longer and doesn't alter the taste of food like plastic can.

TUMMY TAMER

When buying any kind of kitchen equipment, look for the NSF-certified quality label. National Sanitation Foundation (NSF) products undergo safety and quality controls to receive the certification.

The Least You Need to Know

- Use herbs and spices rather than oil when flavoring dishes.
- Avoid spicy, acidic, and hot types of flavorings to help prevent reflux incidents.
- If possible, choose fresh herbs and spices over dry ones for maximum flavor.
- Choose baking, grilling, broiling, and steaming as acid reflux–friendly cooking methods rather than frying, deep-frying, and other methods that use lots of oil.

Chapter 9

Eating Out with Acid Reflux

In This Chapter

- General eating out options
- Making sense of menus
- What's safe to eat where

Eating out is part of life for many people. For some, it's almost required due to work obligations. For others, it is a way to socialize and catch up with family and friends. Even those eating at home may rely on take-out options due to overly booked schedules and lack of time left for cooking, dislike for anything kitchen related, or a simple love of the taste and flavor of take-out options.

Eating out can be part of a healthy diet. Whether you eat out once a year or consume three meals a day from take-out establishments, this chapter equips you with the information you need to enjoy your dining out lifestyle without triggering your acid reflux symptoms.

Before You Go

Before you head out to eat, keep in mind a few points that will make the meal (and afterward) much easier on you. First, look at the restaurant menu ahead of time (many restaurants post menus online these days), and review the choices available to you.

When you see something you like, call ahead and ask if the restaurant is flexible with ingredient substitutions and menu-item modifications. It might help to explain you have acid reflux and can't tolerate some ingredients.

Eat before you head out. This may sound counterintuitive, but having a small snack before heading out can help you avoid succumbing to temptations. One hard-boiled egg with some fruit is a great snack. A handful of nuts with a small fat-free yogurt is another good alternative.

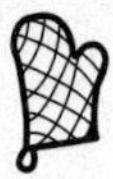

COOLER TALK

Before you head out for a dinner with friends, family, or a loved one, visit menupages.com to preselect what you're going to have. Planning ahead will take the stress off when you're forced to make a decision about your food choices on the spot.

Decoding the Restaurant Menu

Even with your best intentions and sleuthing skills, you still might find terms on menus that you don't understand or are hard to decipher. Use the following guide to identify some terms to avoid:

Au gratin Foods that have a crusted top. They're generally coated with breadcrumbs and a high-fat sauce and then passed under a broiler to create the crust.

Béchamel The butter, flour, and seasonings in this sauce make it too high in fat for those with acid reflux.

Beurre blanc Translated from French, this means "white butter." You'll often see this on vegetables or fish. These dishes are high in fat and can trigger acid reflux.

Bisque This is a cream-based soup. Opt for broth-based varieties instead of cream based to cut down on the fat and calories. Your stomach and your waistline will thank you!

Confit This term designates meat or poultry that's cooked and preserved in its own fat and served hot.

Coupe This ice-cream sundae with fruit on top can be good or bad, depending on whether the ice cream is low fat and what type of fruit is used. In general, it's probably too high in fat for acid reflux sufferers.

Court bouillon Stock containing vinegar or white wine.

Ganache A thick mixture of chocolate and whipped cream used in desserts. Ganache cookies and cakes frequently decorate holiday tables. The chocolate and fat in this dish are the acid reflux triggers.

Rillette This cold mixture of meat or poultry is cooked, mashed, and preserved in its own fat. It's high in fat.

Shortened cake You can translate this as "made with fat."

That's what you should avoid. But what's left? Plenty! Look for grilled, broiled, baked, poached, and steamed dishes. Berries for dessert can be great.

TUMMY TAMER

If you're sensitive to berries, you may consider stashing some plain fat-free yogurt sweetened with a little brown sugar and cinnamon in your office or car (in a freezer bag) so you can have it after your meal without feeling like you're missing out on dessert.

At the Restaurant

The menu offers so many options. When you're hungry, everything sounds good. But before you order something you'll regret, remember the list of no-nos in the preceding section and take another look at the menu, keeping your stomach in mind.

Consider starting your meal with a broth-based soup such as chicken noodle. A cup of warm soup may take the edge off your hunger and soothe your stomach—and prevent overeating later in the meal.

Look at what diners around you are eating. If their portions look too big for you, ask your waiter to doggie bag half of your entrée before bringing it out. Or consider asking for a child's size.

Consider ordering an appetizer as an appetizer and another appetizer as your main course.

A salad can be a great appetizer or main course. Read the list of ingredients carefully and ask your waiter to remove any acid reflux triggers. Ask for the dressing to be served on the side. Better yet, drizzle a little bit of olive oil on your salad and only use the minimum amount necessary to add flavor.

If a tempting treat lands on your table, follow a three-bite rule. Have three small bites, and leave the rest behind.

If you're having a burger or a sandwich that's way too big, take off the top bun and enjoy it as an open sandwich. Alternatively, have half of your portion and save the second half for your next meal. This both decreases the size of your meal, helping with reflux symptoms, and reduces your calorie intake.

ACID ALERT

Craving a burger? That's fine, but remember to avoid the onions, mustard, ketchup, and mayonnaise often added. And avoid making your burger a cheeseburger.

If ordering egg whites at a diner or take-out place, request that your dish be prepared using cooking spray instead of oil. If no spray is available, ask for the least amount of oil.

Instead of focusing on the foods you should *not* eat, think about the abundance of foods you can and should enjoy! Eating is about more than just food. Slow down, and put down your fork between bites. Look around, appreciate the ambiance of the restaurant, and enjoy your company.

Chinese Food

Chinese food can be part of a healthy diet. The two main concerns when it comes to Chinese cuisine are fat and sodium. Opt for steamed dishes and broth-based soups, or order your food with the least amount of oil possible.

The following table gives you more tips for what to eat and what not to eat at Chinese restaurants.

Safe Bets	Foods to Avoid
Wonton soup	Fried wontons
Steamed dumplings	Fried dumplings
Brown rice	Fried rice
Steamed shrimp, meat, or poultry	Pan-fried fish
Vegetable/chicken soong (chopped vegetables/chicken wrapped in lettuce leaves)	Spareribs

Japanese Food

As a dietitian, I could dine in Japanese restaurants on a nightly basis and never get tired of the wide selection of healthy dishes on the menu. As with Chinese food, though, extra added sodium and fat in some dishes is a concern.

Use low-sodium soy sauce, and dip your rolls fish side down—that's the way people in Japan eat them to avoid extra sauce soaking into the rice. Perfect your skills at using chopsticks, too! This can slow down the pace of your meal.

The following table gives you more do's and don'ts for Japanese restaurants.

Safe Bets	Foods to Avoid
Miso soup	Tempura dishes
Edamame (without salt)	Goyza (fried dumplings)
Steamed veggies	Crunch rolls
Fish and veggie sushi	Creamy sauces
Rolls wrapped in cucumber	
Sashimi	
Steamed rice	

Mexican Food

Mexican food can be healthy, as long as you avoid the trigger foods listed in the following table.

If none of the safe-bet dishes are available, examine the other dishes on the menu and identify items from those dishes you can eat. If you see a salad topped with chicken and some sort of dish that has steamed vegetables in it, you know those ingredients are available in the kitchen. Ask your waiter to make a platter of grilled protein and steamed veggies for you.

Safe Bets	Foods to Avoid
Vegetarian black beans	Refried beans
Grilled fish and seafood	Nachos supreme
Broth-based soups	Gazpacho
Fish or tacos	Fried taco salad bowl
Fajitas made with shrimp or chicken	Chimichangas

Italian Food

Italian food can be great both for your acid reflux and your waistline! Traditional Italian recipes don't need to go to waste as long as creativity and preparation take priority. Sticking to what you know is safe allows you to enjoy your favorite Italian meals without compromising the taste.

Check out the following table for safe foods at Italian restaurants.

Safe Bets	Foods to Avoid
Grilled seafood	Garlic bread and rolls
Steamed clams	Anything fried
Grilled chicken or fish	Marinara sauce
Vegetables without garlic	Carbonara sauce
Pasta primavera without sauce	Parmesan dishes
Pizza (whole-wheat crust, little cheese, and lots of veggies)	Rich (high-fat) desserts

French Food

If, when you think of French cuisine, you envision creamy and heavy dishes paired with scrumptious cheese platters and decadent desserts, you might be surprised to learn that French restaurants offer many great choices for those with acid reflux.

First, the portions are generally small! Second, the best traditional dish on most French restaurant menus includes a pot of steamed mussels, which are low in calories and high in protein. Just watch what kind of sauce is used for cooking and skip the french fries dipped into mayo instead of ketchup. A lean steak with a baked potato is another good choice.

Check out the following table for more acid reflux–friendly French foods.

Safe Bets	Foods to Avoid
Steamed mussels	French onion soup
Niçoise salad (dressing on the side)	Creamy soups and sauces
Other green salads	Chocolate
Grilled, poached, or steamed fish	Cheese

Safe Bets	Foods to Avoid
Fruit for dessert (no whipped cream)	Crème caramel
	Rich desserts
	Croissants

American Food

When I was trying to decide what foods to put in this category, all types of menu items came to mind, especially when I thought about different regions of the country. The best thing about American cuisine is that it comprises a great combination of various national and international dishes and flavor combinations. There are generally plenty of acid-reflux safe menu items, as the following table shows.

Safe Bets	Foods to Avoid
Salads with olive oil	Salads with bacon and croutons
Broth-based soups	Cream-based soups
Turkey sandwiches on whole-wheat	Cheeseburgers
Roast beef sandwiches on whole-wheat	Grilled cheese
Grilled fish	French fries
Grilled poultry	Fried dishes
Grilled meat	Reuben sandwiches
Sirloin steak	Milkshakes
Baked potatoes	Juices
Angel food cake	Rich cookies and cakes
Cantaloupe with cottage cheese	

Fast Food

Believe it or not, fast food can be your friend when you're menu planning for acid reflux. As the demand for healthier options has been growing and calorie-labeling regulations in many states have exposed the most caloric- and fat-loaded offenders, fast-food establishments have been responding with a greater selection of healthy options.

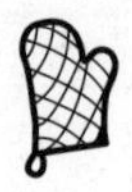

COOLER TALK

Fast food isn't a twentieth-century idea. It actually traces back to ancient Rome, where street vendors sold ready-to-eat food.

If your state doesn't require calories to be labeled on menus just yet, consider going to the restaurant's website and preselecting your choices before you get there. For instance, a bagel can be a great and acid reflux–friendly food. However, the calories in bagels can range from 200 to more than 600, depending on the size and density. Add some cream cheese, and that bagel might go straight to your thighs or midsection!

The following table gives you other fast-food options.

Safe Bets	Foods to Avoid
Bagel with fat-free cream cheese	Tuna salad
Grilled chicken sandwich	Cream-based soups
Plain burgers	French fries
Turkey sandwiches	Fried foods
Roast beef sandwiches	Salads with bacon and croutons
Chicken fajitas	Mashed potatoes
Fruit and fruit salads	Pizza
Fat-free milk	Ketchup
Fat-free yogurt	Mustard

Here are just some of the acid reflux–friendly items you may enjoy. Adhering to the portion sizes is key because, although many of these items are acid reflux friendly, they may be high in fat. A small amount can satisfy your craving without triggering your pain. As always, maintain a detailed food journal to determine your individual triggers.

At McDonald's, scrambled eggs, side salads, snack-size fruit and walnut salads, fruit and maple oatmeal, fruit and yogurt parfaits, vanilla reduced fat ice cream cones, and strawberry sundaes are some of the acceptable choices. Note that the baked desserts such as pies and cookies are high in fat and should be enjoyed only in moderation.

At Burger King, opt for egg omelets, BK fresh apple fries, hamburgers, cheeseburgers (without mayo, onions, tomatoes, pickles, or mustard), Mott's Harvest applesauce, garden salads, or side salads.

At Wendy's, opt for chopped eggs, hamburger patties without buns (excess calories in one sitting may exacerbate acid reflux), low-fat milk with saltines, spring mix salad greens, apple pecan chicken salads, garden salads, Caesar salads, or plain baked potatoes with reduced-fat sour cream. Note that the hamburger is high in fat. Ask for salad dressings on the side, or add a little olive oil instead.

At Au Bon Pain, order apple cinnamon oatmeal or an egg on a bagel with ham. Fresh fruits, mixed nuts, muesli, Turkish apricots, or blueberry, strawberry, or vanilla yogurt with blueberries are also good. Other great choices include cinnamon crisp, honey nine-grain, plain, plain skinny, poppy, or whole-wheat skinny bagels.

At Starbucks, Hawaiian bagels or plain bagels are great when topped with low-fat or fat-free cream cheese. The selection of low-fat yogurts and dairy is wonderful to pair with your bagel for additional protein. Starbucks oatmeal is always a great option. Starbucks parfaits are another good choice for those who can tolerate small amounts of berries. A heads-up, though: these parfaits also contain cardamom and nutmeg if those are on your avoid list.

At Subway, select nine-grain bread, light English muffins, flatbreads, honey Italian bread, or honey oat bread as your base. Fill your sandwich with lean turkey, chicken, or egg whites and top with lettuce, cucumbers, and olives.

At Dunkin Donuts, blueberry, multigrain, plain, and wheat bagels are good choices. A reduced-fat blueberry muffin paired with fat-free milk makes a good mini-meal.

TUMMY TAMER

If you love bagels but your store sells them in huge sizes, consider having ¼ of a large bagel at a time or scooping out the inside and spreading on a thin layer of fat-free cream cheese, light butter, or peanut butter for flavor.

The Least You Need to Know

- Doing some research before departing for the restaurant can save you time and tummy trouble later.
- Ask the waiter to doggie bag half of your entrée if it's too big for you to comfortably eat in one meal.

- Slow down and enjoy the atmosphere and your friends. You'll eat less and enjoy the experience that much more!
- Select acid reflux–friendly choices when dining out, and focus on the abundance of foods you can have instead of those you cannot.

Reflux-Friendly Travel and Social Occasions

Chapter 10

In This Chapter

- Packing pointers
- Avoiding trouble at the airport
- When in Rome …
- Tips for dealing with social situations

If you dread vacation or business trips because you know you could be at the mercy of your acid reflux the entire time, this chapter is for you. In most cases, traveling isn't stressful, but you may look at it as exactly that. Simple precautions such as showing up early and skipping a pretransit fast-food binge can make for a smooth flight. Whether your destination is 300 or 3,000 miles away, this chapter gives you the tools to enjoy your trip free of acid reflux symptoms.

Holidays, parties, and other social situations present their own set of challenges. Many of these occasions are filled with treats that may be difficult to resist—and food pushers who may be adding to the temptation to grab the wrong food. Preparing for such situations ahead of time can make you a natural socialite, confidently handling any difficult predicament that arises.

Before You Leave Home

The best way to prevent something is to stop it before it starts. Easier said than done, right? Well, first things first. You need to become familiar with what triggers your symptoms if you haven't already. This may take a little trial and error, so if you haven't already been keeping a food journal, do so for a few days or weeks prior to your trip. This can help you identify your triggers.

Pack Smart

Although the severity and source of your acid reflux is specific to you, some general tips can help you enjoy a pain-free trip.

First, now is not the time to suffer for fashion. Be sure what you're wearing during transit (and your stay) doesn't have a tight waistband or require a belt. Anything putting pressure on your abdomen will, in turn, loosen the LES valve and could trigger your symptoms. On the bright side, this can be the perfect excuse for why you've kept those "safety pants" all these years.

Don't forget your meds! Especially during long travel times, you want to be as prepared as possible. You may even consider packing some in your carry-on in case your luggage doesn't make it to the final destination.

Elevating your head during sleep is always a good way to control your reflux, but it can get a little tricky when you're away from home. Consider your sleeping arrangements and bring along a neck pillow or even a full-length body wedge. This may not be the most ideal piece of luggage, but that pillow and those 6 inches may become your best friend.

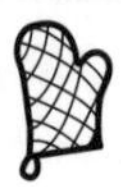

COOLER TALK

The combination of not eating 2 hours before sleep and elevating your head while sleeping gives you 95 percent relief from acid reflux symptoms.

Carry-On Cuisine

Fast eating and overeating are two major contributors that trigger symptoms. You should be eating many small meals throughout each day, so it may be a good idea to bring along your own supply of reflux-friendly foods. This way, you won't have any trouble passing on the in-flight snacks being offered. Here are a few ideas when packing your carry-on:

Fruit:

- Apple, dried
- Apple, fresh
- Banana
- Unsweetened applesauce

Vegetables:

- Baby carrots
- Celery
- Cucumbers, diced

Dairy:

- Cheese, feta or goat
- Soy cheese, low fat

Grains:

- Bread, multigrain or white
- Cereal, bran or oatmeal
- Graham crackers
- Pretzels
- Rice cakes

Sweets/desserts:

- Cookie, fat free
- Jelly beans
- Potato chips, baked
- Red licorice

Nuts:

- Almonds (12 to 24 nuts or a small handful)
- Cashews (12 to 24 nuts or a small handful)
- Pistachios (small handful)
- Walnuts (small handful)

Tea:

- Chamomile
- Ginger

Even those with normal gastrointestinal function and bowel habits often experience discomfort on vacation. Jet lag, new hotel bathrooms, and the lack of easy access to a nearby bathroom when sightseeing, when combined with unfamiliar foods, may provoke irritable bowel symptoms, diarrhea, or constipation. Bringing your own box of cereal, oatmeal, or even bars you know you can eat may minimize these travel woes. If you're unsure of what foods are acceptable to bring on board, get in touch with the airline to see if it has certain restrictions.

At the Airport

Let's face it. Airports (and flying in general) can be stressful. And you know stress is one of the triggers you should avoid if you suffer from acid reflux. Be sure to give yourself ample time for check-in and a little relaxation before takeoff. No matter how familiar you may be with a particular airport, you can never be sure things are running smoothly and on time when you arrive.

After you pass through the security checkpoints, stock up on fluids for your trip. Water is always the best option, but fat-free milk also works. You can sip on it before returning to your waiting area, or pack it away with the rest of the discomfort-free food you've stored for the flight.

If you have a little time on your hands before boarding and you're not interested in sitting still, feel free to stroll down the terminal and see what's available, but keep your list of foods to avoid handy. Although airports are starting to offer more nutritious options, it can be very easy to go for old favorites such as a large frozen coffee drink or an order of french fries. Remember, these choices are full of your worst enemies. Stay away from all the caffeine and fatty food offerings that line the terminals.

Now's also a good time to stock up on gum, if you don't have any on you. Not only does chewing gum help your ears pop as you ascend into the sky, but it also helps your digestion by stimulating the production of saliva, which neutralizes excess stomach acid.

For those of you tempted at the sight of an alcoholic beverage either before or during a flight—beware! Although some people can get away with a few drinks and not experience symptoms, if your reflux becomes more active after drinking, just say no. If you must indulge yourself, stay away from carbonated choices such as beer and champagne. The safest route would be to dilute liquor with water.

TUMMY TAMER

If your flight has been delayed, take some of this time to walk around and allow any food or drink you've consumed to properly digest. After all, you have the whole flight to be confined to a seat.

You're Here! Now What?

Whether you've traveled to the state next door or halfway around the world, now is not the time to let down your guard and indulge in foods you shouldn't eat or activities you've learned will cause problems.

Try to keep your stress levels down. It may be hard to stay focused with any craziness you encounter upon arrival, especially if you've traveled to a foreign country you're not familiar with, but you have to keep your eyes on the prize. It may be necessary to find a happy medium that recognizes and accepts traditions and customs without discounting your needs. Traveling to a foreign country can be stressful enough without the added burden of controlling your reflux. So relax, take a deep breath, and remember what you've learned in previous chapters about what to avoid.

If you didn't already familiarize yourself with the typical lifestyle or traditional foods in the country you're visiting, that should be one of your first tasks. It's important to identify any common ingredients, preparation methods, or styles of dining that may become a potential problem and try to avoid them if possible. For example, if you're visiting coastal regions of Central or South America, be aware that citrus is a common ingredient in many of their dishes such as *ceviche*. In Russia, mayonnaise and lots of fat dominate many dishes. In Spain, a normal day usually consists of several social gatherings that typically involve drinking and tapas well into the night. Plan accordingly to avoid any reflux!

DEFINITION

Ceviche is a dish typically made from fresh raw fish marinated in citrus juices such as lemon or lime and spiced with chile peppers. Additional seasonings such as onion, salt, and pepper may also be added.

Unfortunately, no matter how hard you try, you may still find yourself in a state of discomfort that happens to be completely unavoidable. Don't panic! Fortunately, you should have access to a pharmacy nearby and all you need to do is ask. If a language barrier is a problem, check out the phrases in the following table.

Language	"Where Is the Pharmacy?"
Dutch	"Waar is de apotheek?"
French	"Où est la pharmacie?"
German	"Wo ist die Apotheke?"
Italian	"Doveè la farmacia?"
Russian	"Gde apteka?"
Spanish	"¿Dónde está la farmacia?"

ACID ALERT

Coffee and after-dinner mints can be two reflux triggers. Instead, opt for chamomile tea and enjoy it with licorice candy. Both have been shown to soothe the stomach and alleviate reflux symptoms.

Handling Challenging Social Situations

Dealing with acid reflux in the presence of your family, friends, colleagues, or even a stranger has the potential to create an awkward situation. Remember, when you're in social situations, the rules haven't changed. You still need to take the same precautions as you do at home.

Dealing with Dinner

Meals tend to be the common denominator in a lot of celebrations, family get-togethers, dinner parties, and business meetings. Just because you're out and about, don't forget what you've learned when it comes to foods you can and can't eat. Also, be mindful of the time your meal is taking place. If you want any shot at getting a good night's sleep, remember to follow the no-eating-before-bed-for-2-or-3-hours rule.

Some menus either contain such little information or may be too complicated that you feel like there's no chance of cracking the code on your own. This isn't the time to be shy. Ask any questions you have about the menu. If it helps, remember that you are the paying customer. Reread the restaurant guide in Chapter 9 before heading out, and inform your server of your concerns when it comes time to order. He or she should be more than willing to guide you through the menu.

TUMMY TAMER

While you're looking at the menu, pick out three items you feel are reflux friendly. Compare each of those dishes in terms of flavor, content, and portion size. Now you can choose what to order with complete confidence.

Portion size is essential to keeping your reflux under control. If you know that leaving half of your entrée for later is an unlikely option, consider ordering an appetizer instead.

Be assertive. Don't let close friends and family aid in your downfall. Stick to your guns and don't be persuaded to "try a little of this." Remind your family and friends that you won't be able to enjoy the rest of your night if you decide to give in, even if you're just headed for bed.

If dining at a friend's house, consider bringing your own dish for all to share. The host will appreciate your thoughtfulness, and you won't spend the night hungry. (If you're worried this might hurt your hostess's feelings, you might call ahead and explain your situation.)

Preparing for Parties

Going to a party is very similar to attending a sit-down dinner, only this time there is a greater chance that you will be standing or walking around. Because your body is in the optimal position for digestion, minor reflux symptoms may be less noticeable. You should still avoid certain foods and time your meals to avoid discomfort later, especially when the party takes place during evening and/or nighttime hours.

Many parties serve some sort of alcohol. If you experience reflux symptoms after drinking alcohol, stay away. As previously mentioned, pick your poison carefully, and be sure to limit the amount you consume.

Social Comebacks

You've probably met them: food pushers or well-meaning relatives who simply don't understand your acid reflux symptoms and why you have to restrict your diet. Dealing with them can be stressful.

Practicing a few responses or comebacks can give you confidence to explain your dietary restrictions without sounding defensive or making the situation uncomfortable. Try these, or create a few of your own:

- "I had dinner before I got here, but I would love to take some home for later."
- "I will definitely try this later. I am trying to leave room for the delicious dinner!"
- "The food was amazing. I am so full that I cannot possibly take another bite."

The Least You Need to Know

- Pack acid reflux–friendly snacks when you travel, and leave your acid reflux symptoms behind.
- Learn about traditions and types of cuisine prior to visiting a new country, and you'll save yourself and your tummy a load of trouble.
- If limited food options are available, stick to small portion sizes, slow down while eating your meals, and avoid alcohol and spices.
- If you have an arsenal of polite social comebacks about your diet or acid reflux before heading out to a party, you won't be caught off guard defending your choices again.

Part 4

Recipes for Reflux-Free Living

If you think you'll only be eating bland and unpalatable foods on an acid reflux diet, think again! Part 4 is filled with tons of great recipe ideas that not only soothe your stomach but keep your family happy as well.

If you're new to cooking, don't worry. All the recipes in this book use easy-to-find ingredients and only require a few steps to make. If you're an experienced cook, you can use these recipes as a jumping-off point and brainstorm your own ideas for different flavor combinations.

To make things even easier, many of the recipes can be prepared in bulk and frozen for later quick-reheat meals. Keeping cakes and baggies of cookies in the freezer can prepare you for any unexpected guests and turn you into a favorite host ready to entertain within minutes.

Chapter 11

Good-Start Breakfasts

In This Chapter

- Delicious yogurt treats
- Superb breakfast smoothies
- Protein-packed egg dishes
- Other morning yummies

Breakfast is the most important meal of the day. Starting your day with the right breakfast is a very important step in your daily routine. Having a nutritious breakfast can also set a positive tone for the rest of the day.

The most frequent excuses for skipping breakfast include a lack of time, boredom with the current meal selection, and reflux symptoms after eating some breakfast favorites. Fortunately, this chapter is filled with delicious recipes that take minutes to prepare and leave your stomach feeling comfortable for hours!

Berry Graham Cracker Parfait

Parfaits bring the fun back to yogurt! You'll love starting your day with layers of juicy fruit, creamy yogurt, and crunchy crackers.

Yield:	**Prep time:**	**Serving size:**
2 parfaits	5 minutes	1 parfait
Each serving has:		
180 calories	30 g carbohydrates	2 g fat
4 g fiber	12 g protein	

1 cup fat-free Greek yogurt
1 TB. honey
½ tsp. ground flaxseeds
½ cup fresh blackberries
½ cup fresh blueberries
¼ cup graham cracker crumbs

1. In a small bowl, combine Greek yogurt, honey, and ground flaxseeds.
2. In 2 (8-ounce) cups, layer yogurt mixture with blackberries, blueberries, and graham cracker crumbs.

Variation: For another tasty parfait, consider substituting an equal amount of granola for the graham cracker crumbs.

TUMMY TAMER

Berries are an acid reflux trigger for some people. If they are for you, substitute bananas or an equal amount of canned, unsweetened pumpkin purée instead.

Nutty Greek Yogurt

Salty and crunchy nuts pair nicely with creamy yogurt and sweet agave in this decadent dish.

Yield:	**Prep time:**	**Serving size:**
2 yogurts	5 minutes	1 yogurt
Each serving has:		
340 calories	33 g carbohydrates	14 g fat
9 g fiber	22 g protein	

$1\frac{1}{2}$ cups fat-free *Greek yogurt*

2 TB. agave nectar

$\frac{1}{2}$ cup shelled pistachio nuts

1. In a medium bowl, combine Greek yogurt, agave nectar, and pistachio nuts.
2. Divide between 2 (8-ounce) containers, and serve.

Variation: Honey works beautifully in this recipe instead of agave. Substitute an equal amount of any type of honey for variety.

DEFINITION

Greek yogurt is a strained yogurt, and it's a good natural source of protein, calcium, and probiotics. On average, Greek yogurt contains 40 percent more protein per ounce than traditional yogurt.

Power Breakfast Smoothie

This smoothie is a favorite with kids. It's sweet thanks to the fruit and is an excellent way to sneak in some veggies and calcium.

Yield:	**Prep time:**	**Serving size:**
2 smoothies	5 minutes	1 smoothie
Each serving has:		
153 calories	34 g carbohydrates	0 g fat
4 g fiber	6 g protein	

2 medium bananas, peeled and roughly chopped

2 cups fresh spinach, roughly chopped

1 medium red delicious apple, skin on, cored, and roughly chopped

1 cup skim milk

1. In a blender, combine bananas, spinach, apple, and skim milk, and blend until smooth.
2. Divide between 2 glasses, and serve.

Variation: You can substitute other apple varieties without altering the taste.

ACID ALERT

Protein powders and drinks have gained popularity in recent years, but many have ingredients that may trigger acid reflux symptoms. Make your own yummy, acid reflux–friendly smoothies and shakes instead!

Banana Turmeric Smoothie

This smoothie is sweet, slightly spicy, and delightfully decadent.

Yield: 2 smoothies	**Prep time:** 2 minutes	**Serving size:** 1 smoothie
Each serving has:		
173 calories	36 g carbohydrates	3 g fat
4 g fiber	2 g protein	

2 medium bananas, peeled and roughly chopped

2 cups unsweetened almond milk

½ tsp. ground turmeric

1 tsp. vanilla extract

1. In a blender, combine bananas, almond milk, ground turmeric, and vanilla extract, and blend until smooth.
2. Divide between 2 glasses, and serve.

Variation: During hot summer days, you can add 4 to 6 ice cubes to this recipe to make a cool treat.

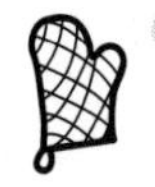

COOLER TALK

Turmeric has been shown to be a natural fat-burner. Add it to many recipes. It goes well with both sweet and savory foods.

Strawberry-Papaya Smoothie

Sweet strawberries and the tropical flavor of papaya will have you coming back for more.

Yield:	**Prep time:**	**Serving size:**
1 smoothie	5 minutes	1 smoothie
Each serving has:		
130 calories	26 g carbohydrates	1.5 g fat
5 g fiber	4 g protein	

1 cup diced ripe papaya

¼ cup plain nonfat yogurt

4 large frozen strawberries

1. In a blender, combine papaya, yogurt, and strawberries.
2. Blend until smooth.

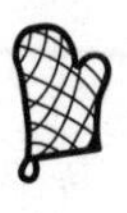

COOLER TALK

This recipe was published in *101 Optimal Life Foods* by David Grotto, RD, LDN. The original recipe was developed by Veronica "Roni" Noone (greenlitebites.com).

Quick Pumpkin Smoothie

A creamy blend of sweet, rich flavors, this vanilla-y, pumpkin-y smoothie will be a great addition to your menu.

Yield:	**Prep time:**	**Serving size:**
1 smoothie	5 minutes	1 smoothie
Each serving has:		
230 calories	42 g carbohydrates	2 g fat
5 g fiber	12 g protein	

½ cup canned pumpkin

½ cup vanilla nonfat yogurt

⅓ cup vanilla soy milk

½ tsp. pumpkin pie spice

2 or 3 ice cubes

1 tsp. agave syrup

1. In a blender, combine canned pumpkin, vanilla yogurt, vanilla soy milk, pumpkin pie spice, ice cubes, and agave syrup.
2. Blend until smooth.

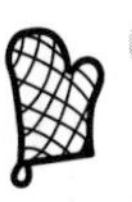

COOLER TALK

This recipe was published in *101 Optimal Life Foods* by David Grotto, RD, LDN. The original recipe was developed by Veronica "Roni" Noone (greenlitebites.com).

Yummy Breakfast Squash

You'll love the sweetness of this butternut squash paired with fresh cottage cheese and the slight crunch of slivered almonds.

Yield:	**Prep time:**	**Cook time:**	**Serving size:**
2 squash halves	5 minutes	10 minutes	1 squash half
Each serving has:			
250 calories	42 g carbohydrates	4 g fat	6 g fiber
18 g protein			

1 medium butternut squash
1 cup fat-free cottage cheese
2 TB. slivered almonds
1 TB. brown sugar, firmly packed
¼ tsp. ground cinnamon

1. Slice butternut squash in half lengthwise, and scoop out and discard seeds.
2. Place squash skin side up on a microwave-safe plate, and microwave on high for 10 minutes or until fork-tender.
3. Fill each squash half with ½ cup cottage cheese. Top with slivered almonds, sprinkle with brown sugar and ground cinnamon, and serve.

Variation: If you don't have almonds, this recipe works great with ground flaxseeds, chopped walnuts, or other nut varieties. No nuts? Skip them altogether—it'll still taste great.

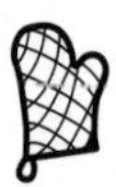

COOLER TALK

Butternut squash is high in vitamin C, calcium, vitamin E, beta-carotene, folate, and potassium.

Asparagus Frittata

Cumin brings excitement and lots of flavor to this old-time breakfast favorite, while asparagus adds a dose of color and slight crunch.

Yield:	**Prep time:**	**Cook time:**	**Serving size:**
1 (9-inch) frittata	5 minutes	30 minutes	1/6 frittata
Each serving has:			
138 calories	4 g carbohydrates	7 g fat	1 g fiber
13 g protein			

3 large eggs

8 large egg whites

1 TB. chopped fresh parsley

1/4 cup fat-free shredded mozzarella cheese

1/4 tsp. salt

1 TB. vegetable oil

3 chicken tenders, cut into 1-in. strips

1/2 tsp. ground cumin

8 asparagus spears, chopped

1. Preheat the oven to 350°F.
2. In a medium bowl, whisk together eggs and egg whites. Add parsley, mozzarella cheese, and salt, and whisk again to combine. Set aside.
3. In a 9-inch oven-proof skillet over high heat, heat vegetable oil. Add chicken strips and ground cumin, and cook, stirring occasionally, for 2 or 3 minutes or until chicken turns golden brown on all sides.
4. Pour egg mixture over chicken, and top with asparagus.
5. Bake *frittata* for 20 minutes. Allow to cool before serving.

DEFINITION

A **frittata** is a skillet-cooked mixture of eggs and other ingredients that's not stirred but cooked slowly and then either flipped or finished under the broiler. This version skips the flipping and the broiling, while still producing an equal amount of flavor.

Breakfast Strata

Spinach, shiitake mushrooms, and cheese add incredible flavor to this strata, while eggs and turkey provide the sustenance that will leave you full for hours.

Yield:	**Prep time:**	**Cook time:**	**Serving size:**
1 (8×8-inch) strata	10 minutes	30 minutes	¼ strata
Each serving has:			
207 calories	20 g carbohydrates	2 g fat	4 g fiber
29 g protein			

8 slices light bread (45 calories or less per slice)

½ cup fat-free ricotta cheese

8 slices thinly sliced low-sodium baked turkey breast

½ cup shiitake mushrooms, roughly chopped

1 cup fresh spinach, roughly chopped

1 (15-oz.) pkg. liquid egg whites

½ cup fat-free shredded mozzarella cheese

1. Preheat the oven to 350°F. Spray an 8×8-inch baking pan with nonstick cooking spray.
2. Place 4 slices of bread in a single layer in the prepared baking pan. Top with ricotta cheese and turkey breast, followed by mushrooms and spinach. Top with remaining 4 slices of bread, and pour egg whites over all, followed by mozzarella cheese.
3. Bake *strata* for 30 minutes. Cool for about 5 minutes, slice into 4 squares, and serve.

Variation: If you like other mushroom varieties, use your favorites instead. Not a fan of spinach? Try an equal amount of steamed broccoli instead.

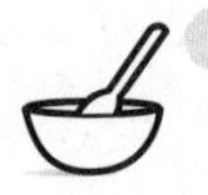

DEFINITION

A **strata** is a savory bread pudding made with eggs and cheese.

Cheese, Spinach, and Avocado Omelet

The freshness of vegetables pairs nicely with the richness of feta cheese to produce a filling breakfast staple.

Yield:	**Prep time:**	**Cook time:**	**Serving size:**
1 omelet	5 minutes	5 minutes	1 omelet
Each serving has:			
325 calories	6 g carbohydrates	26 g fat	3 g fiber
19 g protein			

1 large egg

2 large egg whites

$\frac{1}{8}$ tsp. salt

1 TB. olive oil

2 medium white mushrooms, chopped

$\frac{1}{2}$ cup chopped fresh spinach

$\frac{1}{4}$ medium avocado, peeled, seeded, and thinly sliced

2 TB. reduced-fat crumbled feta cheese

1. In a small bowl, whisk together egg, egg whites, and salt. Set aside.
2. Add olive oil to a small skillet, and set over medium heat. When hot, add mushrooms, and cook for 1 minute. Add spinach, and cook for 1 or 2 more minutes or until spinach is wilted. Remove spinach and mushrooms from the skillet, and set aside.
3. Pour egg mixture into the skillet, and cook for about 1 minute. Tilt the skillet to cook uncooked portions of egg mixture.
4. Add avocado, spinach, and mushrooms to one side of cooked eggs, top with feta cheese, and cook for 1 more minute.
5. Using a spatula, flip untopped side of eggs over spinach and mushrooms. Reduce heat to medium-low, and cook for 1 or 2 more minutes or until eggs are cooked through. Serve *omelet* immediately.

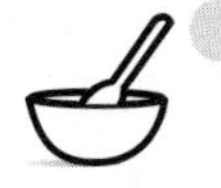

DEFINITION

An **omelet** is usually a morning dish made of beaten eggs that are cooked until set. It's often folded and has a filling such as meat, vegetables, or cheese.

Spinach Egg Muffin

Goat cheese has an intense flavor that pairs very well with the spinach and eggs in this recipe.

Yield: 2 muffins	**Prep time:** 2 minutes	**Cook time:** 5 minutes	**Serving size:** 1 muffin
Each serving has:			
371 calories	29 g carbohydrates	21 g fat	5 g fiber
20 g protein			

1 TB. olive oil

3 cups fresh spinach

2 large eggs

2 whole-wheat English muffins, toasted

$\frac{1}{2}$ cup crumbled goat's milk cheese

1. Place olive oil in a small skillet, and set over high heat. When hot, add spinach, and cook for about 2 minutes or until wilted. Remove spinach to a small plate, and set aside.
2. Add eggs to the skillet, and cook to your desired degree of doneness. Place 1 egg each onto 2 English muffin halves.
3. Top with spinach and goat's milk cheese, top with remaining 2 English muffin halves, and serve.

TUMMY TAMER

If you're concerned about your cholesterol, substitute 2 egg whites for the 1 egg in this recipe.

Egg Scramble

Potatoes bring comfort to this eggy breakfast dish, while rosemary adds a punch of flavor.

Yield:	Prep time:	Cook time:	Serving size:
1 scramble	15 minutes	40 minutes	½ scramble
Each serving has:			
223 calories 19 g protein	13 g carbohydrates	11 g fat	2 g fiber

1 medium Yukon Gold potato
½ tsp. salt
2 large eggs
4 large egg whites
¼ cup fat-free shredded mozzarella cheese
1 TB. light butter
2 TB. chopped fresh rosemary

1. In a small saucepan, place potato and salt. Fill the pan with water. Set over high heat, and bring to a boil. Reduce heat to medium, and boil for about 20 minutes or until potato is fork-tender.
2. When potato is cool enough to handle, dice into ½-inch cubes. Set aside.
3. In a medium bowl, beat eggs and egg whites. Add mozzarella cheese, and stir. Set aside.
4. In a small skillet over high heat, heat light butter. When hot, add diced potatoes and rosemary, and cook, stirring frequently, for about 5 minutes or until potatoes are golden brown.
5. Add egg mixture to potatoes, and cook, stirring frequently, for about 5 minutes or until eggs are done.
6. Divide into 2 portions, and serve warm.

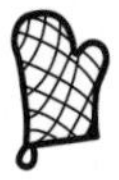

COOLER TALK

A medium potato has more potassium than a banana. Be sure to eat yours with the skin on to get an added dose of fiber!

Baked Breakfast Apple

The natural sweetness of apples in this recipe pairs beautifully with the flavor of maple syrup and the crunchiness of added walnuts and granola.

Yield:	**Prep time:**	**Cook time:**	**Serving size:**
2 apples	5 minutes	8 minutes	1 apple
Each serving has:			
300 calories	50 g carbohydrates	9 g fat	6 g fiber
10 g protein			

2 medium apples (your favorite), skin on and cored

4 TB. water

2 TB. maple syrup

¼ tsp. ground cinnamon

½ cup fat-free vanilla Greek yogurt

6 chopped walnuts

4 TB. granola

1. Place apples in a medium microwave-safe bowl with water. Evenly divide maple syrup and cinnamon between centers of cored apples.
2. Microwave for 7 or 8 minutes or until apples are fork-tender.
3. Fill each apple with ¼ cup yogurt and top with 3 chopped walnuts and 2 tablespoons granola.

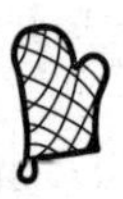

COOLER TALK

Walnuts are a great source of omega-3s, healthy fats, and fiber. Add them to your oatmeal, baked goods, salads, and other dishes. Large amounts of fat may trigger acid reflux symptoms in some, so keep your portions under control and monitor your individual symptoms.

Delicious Quick Breads and Grains

Chapter 12

In This Chapter

- Bountiful breads
- Amazing grains
- Delicious pancakes

There's nothing like the smell of fresh muffins in the oven to make a house smell like a home. This chapter's Apple Walnut Muffins will fill your home with the best aroma and make you count the minutes until you can dig into one of these delightful treats. This recipe not only tastes phenomenal, but it is also incredibly easy to make!

The other breakfast choices in this chapter are equally delicious, nutritious, and fun. Savory oatmeal is filled with soluble fiber, which helps lower your cholesterol, and calcium, which helps prevent osteoporosis. Cottage Cheese Pancakes are filled with calcium, protein, and antioxidants—all of which are nutritional powerhouses. You would never guess any of this because the recipes in this chapter taste so incredible!

Apple Walnut Muffins

Light and slightly sweet, these muffins satisfy a muffin craving without loads of extra calories or added fat.

Yield:	Prep time:	Cook time:	Serving size:
6 muffins	15 minutes	20 minutes	1 muffin
Each serving has:			
238 calories	44 g carbohydrates	4 g fat	2 g fiber
7 g protein			

1¾ cups all-purpose flour
¼ tsp. salt
¾ cup fat-free milk
⅓ cup sugar
¼ cup applesauce
1 tsp. vanilla extract
2 large egg whites
¼ cup finely chopped walnuts
1 medium Granny Smith apple, cored and finely chopped

1. Preheat the oven to 400°F. Spray a 6-cup muffin tin with nonstick cooking spray.
2. In a large bowl, combine all-purpose flour, salt, fat-free milk, sugar, applesauce, vanilla extract, and egg whites. Mix with a spoon or a spatula just until uniformly moist. Fold in walnuts and apple.
3. Spread batter evenly among the 6 prepared muffin cups. Bake for 20 minutes or until muffins are golden-brown on top.
4. Remove from the oven, and cool for a few minutes before serving.

TUMMY TAMER

This recipe is great with almonds or flaxseeds, too! Also try an equal amount of fresh, peeled, and chopped bananas or raisins instead of apples for your next batch.

Nutty Good Millet Muffins

These sweet and nutty muffins are perfect for breakfast or as a snack.

Yield:	**Prep time:**	**Cook time:**	**Serving size:**
12 muffins	10 minutes	15 minutes	1 muffin
Each serving has:			
240 calories	32 g carbohydrates	10 g fat	3 g fiber
2 g protein			

1½ cups whole-wheat flour

¾ cup hazelnut meal or almond meal

½ cup millet

½ tsp. salt

1 TB. baking powder

½ tsp. freshly peeled and grated nutmeg

2 eggs

1 cup buttermilk

⅔ cup plus ¼ cup light brown sugar, firmly packed

6 TB. Earth Balance buttery spread, melted

1 TB. flaxseed meal

1. Preheat the oven to 350°F. Move the rack to the middle of the oven. Line 2 muffin pans with paper liners or spray with nonstick cooking spray.
2. In a small bowl, whisk together whole-wheat flour, ½ cup hazelnut meal, millet, salt, baking powder, and nutmeg. Set aside.
3. In a large bowl, combine eggs, buttermilk, ⅔ cup light brown sugar, and 5 tablespoons melted Earth Balance spread.
4. Add dry ingredients to egg mixture, and fold gently to combine.
5. Drop batter by ice-cream scoops into the muffin pans.
6. In a small bowl, combine remaining ¼ cup light brown sugar, remaining ¼ cup hazelnut meal, flaxseed meal, and remaining 1 tablespoon melted Earth Balance buttery spread. Top each muffin with 1 teaspoon topping, spreading it around to cover top of muffin.
7. Bake for 15 minutes or until a toothpick inserted into the center comes out clean.

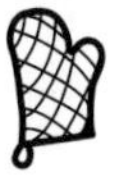

COOLER TALK

This recipe was published in *101 Optimal Life Foods* by David Grotto, RD, LDN. The original recipe was developed by chef Jennifer Carden, author of *The Toddler Café* (thetoddlercafe.blogspot.com).

Basic French Toast

French toast tops the list of comfort foods for many of us. This one delivers a perfect combination of vanilla and cinnamon.

Yield:	**Prep time:**	**Cook time:**	**Serving size:**
4 slices	5 minutes	4 minutes	2 slices
Each serving has:			
237 calories	34 g carbohydrates	4 g fat	1 g fiber
15 g protein			

1 TB. light butter
4 large egg whites
1 tsp. vanilla extract
¼ tsp. ground cinnamon
1 tsp. sugar
½ cup skim milk
4 (½-in.) slices sourdough bread

1. In a large skillet over medium-high heat, heat light butter.
2. Meanwhile, in a medium bowl, whisk together egg whites, vanilla extract, ground cinnamon, sugar, and skim milk.
3. Dip bread slices into egg mixture 1 slice at a time, and transfer to the skillet. Cook for about 2 minutes on each side or until golden brown. Serve 2 slices on each plate.

Variation: This French toast is delicious topped with 1 tablespoon maple syrup per 2 slices or sprinkled with ½ teaspoon confectioners' sugar.

TUMMY TAMER

You can decrease the number of calories in this recipe by wiping the pan with a paper towel before adding the toast. This leaves enough butter to coat the pan while removing excess.

Stuffed French Toast

The slight crunchiness and sweetness on the outside of this French toast pairs nicely with the creaminess of the cream cheese and the sweetness and flavor of the fig inside.

Yield:	**Prep time:**	**Cook time:**	**Serving size:**
2 pieces stuffed toast	5 minutes	6 minutes	1 stuffed toast
Each serving has:			
201 calories	30 g carbohydrates	3.5 g fat	2 g fiber
13 g protein			

1 large egg

3 large egg whites

1 tsp. vanilla extract

¼ tsp. ground cinnamon

½ cup skim milk

½ cup fat-free cream cheese

1 TB. fig jam

4 slices light bread (45 calories or less per slice)

1 TB. light butter

1. In a medium bowl, whisk together egg, egg whites, vanilla extract, ground cinnamon, and skim milk.
2. In a small bowl, combine cream cheese and fig jam.
3. Distribute cream cheese mixture evenly between 2 slices of bread, and top with remaining 2 slices.
4. In a medium skillet over medium-high heat, heat light butter.
5. Dip stuffed toast into egg mixture, turning over to coat both sides evenly. Add stuffed toast to the skillet, and cook for about 3 minutes per side or until bread is golden brown.
6. Serve stuffed toast on a plate.

Variation: For a little something extra, sprinkle with a small amount of confectioners' sugar before serving.

TUMMY TAMER

If you don't have any fig jam, or simply aren't a big fan of figs, substitute ½ a mashed banana or any other jam in this recipe.

Breakfast Power Balls

Better than store-bought granola bars, these fruity power concoctions deliver just the right combination of sweetness and crunch to satisfy both adults and children in the family.

Yield:	Prep time:	Cook time:	Serving size:
24 balls	10 minutes	2 minutes	2 balls
Each serving has:			
90 calories	18 g carbohydrates	2 g fat	1 g fiber
1 g protein			

1 cup chopped dates

1 cup golden raisins

¼ cup unsweetened shredded coconut

¾ cup old-fashioned oats

¼ cup ground flaxseeds

¾ cup white chocolate chips

3 TB. maple syrup

1. In a large bowl, combine dates, golden raisins, shredded coconut, oats, and ground flaxseeds. Set aside.
2. Place white chocolate chips in a microwave-safe container, and microwave on high for about 30 seconds. Remove from the microwave, and stir. If not melted, microwave for another 20 seconds. Repeat until chips are melted and soft.
3. Mix melted chocolate and maple syrup into date mixture. Form mixture into 24 (½-inch) balls, and place them in a separate container. Eat immediately, or refrigerate for later use.

Variation: You can use different types of oats in this recipe. The old-fashioned variety gives it a crunchier taste, whereas instant oatmeal provides a softer texture.

TUMMY TAMER

These little power creations can be frozen in small zipper-lock plastic bags and used as a quick breakfast, a delicious snack, a picnic treat, or a great way to fuel on a long hike.

Homemade Granola

Crunchy and perfectly sweetened, this granola is ideal on its own or as a topping for yogurt or fruit salad.

Yield:	**Prep time:**	**Cook time:**	**Serving size:**
3 cups	10 minutes	$1\frac{1}{2}$ hours	$\frac{1}{4}$ cup
Each serving has:			
122 calories	23 g carbohydrates	3 g fat	2 g fiber
2 g protein			

$\frac{1}{3}$ cup light brown sugar, firmly packed

3 TB. warm water

$\frac{2}{3}$ cup dried cherries

1 TB. unsweetened shredded coconut

2 TB. slivered almonds

1 tsp. vanilla extract

1 TB. ground flaxseeds

2 cups old-fashioned oatmeal

2 TB. agave nectar

$\frac{1}{4}$ tsp. ground cinnamon

1 tsp. all-purpose flour

1 tsp. whole-wheat flour

1 TB. walnut oil

1. Preheat the oven to 220°F. Spray a cookie sheet with nonstick cooking spray.
2. In a large bowl, combine light brown sugar with warm water. Add dried cherries, shredded coconut, slivered almonds, vanilla extract, ground flaxseeds, oatmeal, agave nectar, ground cinnamon, all-purpose flour, whole-wheat flour, and walnut oil, and mix thoroughly.
3. Spread granola mixture on the prepared cookie sheet. Bake for about 90 minutes, mixing granola with a spatula about every 30 minutes to ensure equal cooking.
4. Remove from the oven, and cool prior to serving.

TUMMY TAMER

Granola can make a great on-the-go snack. Pack some in individual bags or small containers, and carry it in your bag. Enjoy in the middle of the day with a cup of chamomile tea.

Tummy Soother Granola

This granola is crunchy, nutty, and slightly sweet.

Yield:	**Prep time:**	**Cook time:**	**Serving size:**
15 servings	10 minutes	30 minutes	$^1/_{15}$ recipe
Each serving has:			
223 calories	27 g carbohydrates	12 g fat	3 g fiber
6 g protein			

3 cups rolled oats

1 cup crystallized ginger, chopped

$^1/_4$ cup shredded coconut

$^1/_4$ cup walnuts

$^1/_4$ cup pumpkin seeds

$^1/_4$ cup flaxseed

$1^1/_2$ tsp. ground cinnamon

1 cup almond or peanut butter

1 tsp. salt (optional if almond or peanut butter is unsalted)

$^3/_4$ cup honey

$^1/_4$ cup water

1. Preheat the oven to 350°F. Spray a glass or metal baking dish with nonstick cooking spray.
2. In the prepared baking dish, combine rolled oats, crystallized ginger, coconut, walnuts, pumpkin seeds, flaxseed, and ground cinnamon. Toast for about 10 minutes.
3. Meanwhile, in a small bowl, combine almond butter, salt (if using), honey, and water.
4. Remove the baking dish from the oven, and mix in almond butter mixture using a spatula. Flatten granola into an even layer.
5. Bake for about 20 minutes. Let cool, and slice into bars or break into clusters.

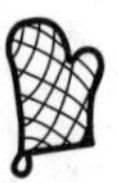

COOLER TALK

This recipe was developed by Ayla Withee, RD, LDN, of Eat Simply Nutrition (eatsimply.org).

Go Nuts for Muesli

This traditional European staple is nutty and crunchy and pairs perfectly with cold milk.

Yield: 3 cups	**Prep time:** 5 minutes	**Serving size:** ½ cup
Each serving has:		
307 calories	36 g carbohydrates	17 g fat
6 g fiber	6 g protein	

1 cup chopped raw hazelnuts, unsalted

¾ cup macadamia nuts

¼ cup unsweetened flaked coconut

1 TB. ground flaxseeds

½ cup chopped dried apples

2½ cups old-fashioned oats

1. In a medium bowl, combine hazelnuts, macadamia nuts, flaked coconut, ground flaxseeds, apples, and old-fashioned oats.
2. Serve with cold milk or yogurt.

TUMMY TAMER

Muesli is a great nutritious food, but it's pretty high in calories. Consider using it as a topping for yogurt or making a muesli parfait. You can also create a complete and satisfying meal by having a portion of muesli and an egg white omelet for breakfast.

Georgia Pecan Muesli

This muesli is perfectly fruity and nutty and goes well with fat-free milk or almond milk or as a yogurt topping.

Yield:	**Prep time:**	**Serving size:**
6 servings	5 minutes	1/6 recipe
Each serving has:		
360 calories	54 g carbohydrates	13 g fat
7 g fiber	8 g protein	

- 2 cups old-fashioned rolled oats
- 1 cup chopped pecans
- 1/2 cup oat bran
- 1/4 cup light brown sugar, firmly packed
- 1/4 cup golden raisins
- 1/4 cup diced dried figs
- 1/4 cup diced dates
- 1/4 tsp. salt

1. In a large bowl, combine rolled oats, pecans, oat bran, light brown sugar, raisins, figs, dates, and salt.
2. Serve with yogurt or milk and fresh fruit, such as banana, if desired.

Variation: For a softer, creamier texture, stir yogurt or milk into the muesli and refrigerate overnight before serving. This is also delicious drizzled with honey.

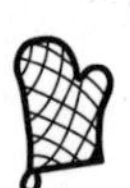

COOLER TALK

This recipe was published in *101 Optimal Life Foods* by David Grotto, RD, LDN. The original recipe was developed by chef Scott Peacock, courtesy of the Georgia Pecan Commission (georgiapecansfit.org).

Fruity Quinoa

Fluffy quinoa combine with the juicy sweetness of dried fruit to create a perfect breakfast staple.

Yield:	**Prep time:**	**Cook time:**	**Serving size:**
2½ cups	5 minutes	15 minutes	½ cup
Each serving has:			
208 calories	41 g carbohydrates	4 g fat	4 g fiber
6 g protein			

1 cup water
1 cup apple juice
1 cup quinoa
¼ cup raisins
¼ cup dried cherries
2 TB. slivered almonds

1. In a medium saucepan over high heat, combine water, apple juice, quinoa, raisins, dried cherries, and almonds. Bring to a boil, reduce heat to medium, cover, and cook for about 15 minutes or until all water is absorbed.
2. Remove from heat and allow to stand for about 5 minutes.
3. Serve in individual small bowls, warm or cold.

Variation: This dish is also delicious cold as a cereal topped with cold soy milk.

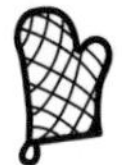

COOLER TALK

Almonds have a long history, dating to 1400 C.E. Today, California is the almond capital, with more than 100,000 acres of land devoted to growing almond trees.

Creamy Cherry Oatmeal

The flavor of cherries pairs nicely with vanilla and brown sugar and adds just the right amount of sweetness to this oatmeal.

Yield:	**Prep time:**	**Cook time:**	**Serving size:**
4 servings	5 minutes	13 minutes	¼ recipe
Each serving has:			
210 calories	35 g carbohydrates	4 g fat	2 g fiber
8 g protein			

2 cups 2 percent milk

1 cup water

1 cup rolled oats

½ cup dried tart cherries

2 tsp. vanilla extract

¼ tsp. ground cinnamon

⅛ tsp. freshly peeled and grated nutmeg

⅛ tsp. salt

1 TB. light brown sugar (firmly packed), honey, or agave syrup

1. In a medium saucepan over medium heat, combine 2 percent milk, water, rolled oats, cherries, vanilla extract, ground cinnamon, nutmeg, salt, and light brown sugar.
2. Simmer, stirring occasionally, for 10 to 13 minutes or until desired creaminess is achieved.

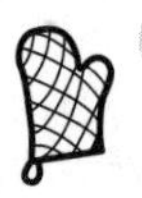

COOLER TALK

This recipe was published in *101 Optimal Life Foods* by David Grotto, RD, LDN. The original recipe was originally developed by Sharon Grotto.

Tropical Oatmeal

Coconut and dates add natural sweetness and tropical undertones to this oatmeal. It's so delicious, you may even consider enjoying it as a snack or dessert.

Yield:	**Prep time:**	**Cook time:**	**Serving size:**
1 cup oatmeal	3 minutes	10 minutes	½ cup oatmeal
Each serving has:			
165 calories	33 g carbohydrates	3 g fat	3 g fiber
3 g protein			

½ cup old-fashioned oats

1 cup unsweetened vanilla almond milk

2 TB. brown sugar, firmly packed

1 TB. toasted coconut

½ medium banana, peeled and chopped

1. In a small saucepan over medium heat, cook oats with almond milk according to the package directions.
2. Mix in brown sugar, toasted coconut, and banana.
3. Serve in 2 small bowls.

ACID ALERT

Coconut is naturally high in fat and may trigger reflux symptoms. Use small amounts in your recipes, and monitor your individual tolerance by keeping a detailed food journal.

Power Oatmeal

Creamy, warm, and slightly sweet, this oatmeal is ideal for a cold winter morning.

Yield: 3 cups	**Prep time:** 5 minutes	**Cook time:** 1 minute	**Serving size:** 1½ cups
Each serving has: 370 calories 8 g protein	59 g carbohydrates	12 g fat	8 g fiber

2 cups unsweetened almond milk

1 cup 1-minute oatmeal

1 TB. ground flaxseeds

2 TB. brown sugar

¼ tsp. ground cinnamon

1 small banana, peeled and finely chopped

1 TB. light butter

1. In a medium saucepan over medium-high heat, bring almond milk to a boil. Add oatmeal, ground flaxseeds, brown sugar, ground cinnamon, and chopped banana. Bring back to a boil, and cook for 1 minute.
2. Remove from heat, add light butter, and stir.
3. Serve warm in 2 bowls.

Variation: If you prefer, you may use skim or soy milk instead of almond milk in this recipe. This substitution provides a creamier texture but also a slight increase in the total calories.

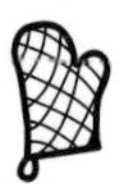

COOLER TALK

Flaxseed is a great addition to your diet. It's high in omega-3 healthy fats, magnesium, phosphorous, copper, thiamin, manganese, and dietary fiber. Add it to soups, salads, baked goods, and yogurts.

Cheesy Oatmeal

Salty, creamy, and cheesy—yes, your morning oatmeal can taste this good!

Yield:	Prep time:	Cook time:	Serving size:
2 cups	1 minute	1 minute	1 cup
Each serving has:			
315 calories 24 g protein	41 g carbohydrates	7 g fat	5 g fiber

- 2 cups skim milk
- 1 cup 1-minute oatmeal
- $\frac{1}{8}$ tsp. salt
- $\frac{1}{2}$ cup fat-free grated mozzarella cheese
- 2 TB. reduced-fat grated Parmesan cheese
- 1 TB. light butter

1. In a medium saucepan over medium-high heat, bring skim milk to a boil. Add oatmeal, salt, $\frac{1}{4}$ cup mozzarella cheese, Parmesan cheese, and light butter, and cook for 1 minute.
2. Serve warm in 2 bowls, sprinkled with remaining $\frac{1}{4}$ cup fat-free mozzarella cheese.

TUMMY TAMER

If you're a vegan, lactose intolerant, or simply looking for variety in your diet, substitute nutritional yeast flakes for the Parmesan cheese in this recipe. You can find nutritional yeast flakes in most supermarkets or online. It's naturally high in vitamin B_{12}, a nutrient lacking in the diets of many vegans.

Cottage Cheese Pancakes

If variety is the spice of life, then these pancakes are the right fit for you. They're slightly browned on the outside, very moist and juicy on the inside, and have a perfect hint of sweetness and spice.

Yield:	**Prep time:**	**Cook time:**	**Serving size:**
4 pancakes	10 minutes	10 minutes	2 pancakes
Each serving has:			
392 calories	57 g carbohydrates	8 g fat	1 g fiber
23 g protein			

1 cup fat-free cottage cheese
2 large eggs
2 TB. sugar
1 TB. maple syrup
$\frac{1}{4}$ tsp. ground cinnamon
$\frac{1}{4}$ tsp. baking powder
$\frac{1}{8}$ tsp. baking soda
$\frac{1}{2}$ cup whole-wheat pastry flour
$\frac{1}{2}$ cup cream of wheat
1 TB. light butter

1. In a large bowl, combine fat-free cottage cheese, eggs, sugar, maple syrup, ground cinnamon, baking powder, baking soda, whole-wheat pastry flour, and cream of wheat.
2. In a large skillet over medium heat, heat light butter. Divide cottage cheese mixture into 4 portions, and place each portion in the skillet. Cook for 5 minutes on one side. Flip over with a spatula, and cook for 5 minutes on the other side.
3. Serve warm, 2 pancakes on a plate.

TUMMY TAMER

These pancakes are a delicious breakfast treat, but two of them contain 23 grams protein, which also makes them a perfect postworkout treat!

Airy Berry Pancakes

A balance of soft texture and fresh taste with a right amount of zest and acidity make these light and airy pancakes a perfect breakfast staple.

Yield:	**Prep time:**	**Cook time:**	**Serving size:**
4 pancakes	10 minutes	10 minutes	1 pancake
Each serving has:			
277 calories	56 g carbohydrates	1 g fat	2 g fiber
12 g protein			

1½ cups cake flour
2 TB. sugar
2 tsp. baking powder
½ tsp. baking soda
2 large egg whites
1 cup nonfat Greek yogurt
¼ cup fat-free buttermilk
1 cup fresh or frozen blueberries

1. In a small bowl, combine cake flour, sugar, baking powder, and baking soda. Add egg whites, Greek yogurt, and fat-free buttermilk. Using an electric hand mixer on medium speed, mix for 1 minute or until smooth.
2. Fold in fresh blueberries.
3. Heat a large skillet over medium heat, and spray with nonstick cooking spray. Separate batter into 4 portions, and cook 2 pancakes at a time for about 3 minutes on each side or until golden brown.
4. Serve with maple syrup or sprinkled with confectioners' sugar.

ACID ALERT

Berries may trigger acid reflux in some people. If they're a trigger for you, substitute bananas in this recipe or skip fruit altogether. It will still come out yummy!

Banana Walnut Waffles

These sweet waffles are complemented by bananas and walnuts for added flavor.

Yield:	Prep time:	Cook time:	Serving size:
5 (3-inch) waffles	15 minutes	5 minutes	1 waffle
Each serving has:			
384 calories	78 g carbohydrates	5 g fat	10 g fiber
13 g protein			

2½ cups whole-wheat flour
⅓ cup light brown sugar, firmly packed
2¼ tsp. baking powder
1 tsp. baking soda
½ tsp. salt
½ cup chopped walnuts
5 egg whites
2 cups low-fat buttermilk
3 ripe medium bananas (with brown spots on the peel)
6 TB. applesauce

1. Preheat a waffle iron, and brush lightly with 2 tablespoons vegetable oil or spray with nonstick cooking spray.
2. In a medium bowl, combine whole-wheat flour, light brown sugar, baking powder, baking soda, salt, and walnuts.
3. In a large bowl, whisk together egg whites, low-fat buttermilk, bananas, and applesauce.
4. Slowly whisk in dry ingredients until well blended.
5. Place 2 cups batter into the waffle iron, and evenly spread batter quickly. Cook based on manufacturer's instructions. Repeat with remaining batter.
6. Serve 1 waffle per plate.

Variation: For a little more sweetness, sprinkle with ¼ teaspoon confectioners' sugar.

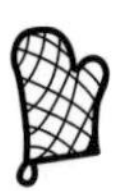

COOLER TALK

Agave nectar has gained popularity due to its relatively low glycemic index compared to other sweeteners. You can use it in tea, smoothies, or baked goods instead of honey or maple syrup.

Banana Crepes with Ricotta Honey

The sweetness of ripe bananas pairs well with the crunchiness of pistachios to add just the right amount of flavor to these crepes.

Yield:	Prep time:	Cook time:	Serving size:
8 crepes	35 minutes	10 minutes	1 crepe
Each serving has:			
112 calories	11 g carbohydrates	6 g fat	3 g fiber
6 g protein			

3 TB. unsweetened applesauce
½ cup low-fat milk
3 large egg whites
½ cup whole-wheat flour
1 tsp. salt
3 TB. honey
3 ripe medium bananas (with brown spots)
1 cup low-fat ricotta cheese
½ cup toasted and chopped pistachios
¼ cup confectioners' sugar

1. In a blender, combine unsweetened applesauce, low-fat milk, egg whites, whole-wheat flour, salt, and 2 tablespoons honey. Cover batter with plastic wrap and refrigerate for 30 minutes or up to 2 days.
2. Heat a medium skillet or crepe pan over medium-high heat. Briefly remove the pan from heat and coat with nonstick cooking spray. Pour ¼ cup batter into the skillet, swirling the pan until batter evenly coats the bottom. Cook for about 2 minutes or until bottom of crepe is golden, flip over crepe, and cook for 10 more seconds. Remove cooked crepe to a plate, and continue with remaining batter.
3. Heat a large skillet over medium-high heat, and spray with nonstick cooking spray. Add bananas, and cook for 2 minutes, turning occasionally, until they're slightly brown.
4. Add remaining 1 tablespoon honey, and cook for 1 more minute. Transfer to a bowl, and cover with aluminum foil.

5. Assemble crepes by placing 1 crepe on a plate. Add a dollop of ricotta cheese in middle of crepe. Add 1 spoonful warm bananas, and top with pistachios. Fold crepe sides over each other so they slightly overlap. Garnish with confectioners' sugar, and serve.

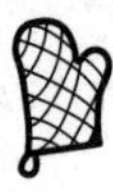

COOLER TALK

The riper the bananas, the sweeter and more alkaline-forming they are. That means they'll help neutralize the acidity and may provide pain relief.

Mouthwatering Snacks and Appetizers

Chapter

13

In This Chapter

- Dips for all occasions
- Delicious finger foods
- Yummy, crowd-pleasing appetizers and snacks

Snacks and appetizers wear many hats. They decorate our tables during holidays, serve as preludes to special meals, and seduce our palates and create special memories on many unforgettable dates. They are also some of the hardest treats to handle for those struggling with acid reflux because many appetizers are coated with fat, butter, tomato sauce, and spices.

Whether you're preparing for a big celebration or just looking for a snack, the recipes in this chapter take all the guesswork out of cooking for you.

Turkey Pinwheels

A little bit of raisins, fresh apples, and dark leafy greens give these small roll-ups an infusion of fresh flavor and a perfect amount of moisture.

Yield:	Prep time:	Serving size:
12 pinwheels	15 minutes	2 pinwheels
Each serving has:		
98 calories	13 g carbohydrates	3 g fat
2 g fiber	7 g protein	

4 medium whole-wheat wraps

4 TB. fat-free cream cheese

1 cup raw spinach

¼ cup raisins

8 slices low-fat, low-sodium turkey breast

½ large apple (your favorite), cored and sliced thin

1. Lay each wrap flat on a work surface, and evenly divide cream cheese among wraps. Add ¼ cup spinach leaves to each wrap, and distribute raisins over each.
2. Add 2 slices turkey to each wrap, and top with thinly sliced apple.
3. Roll up wrap like a burrito, using toothpicks if necessary to hold wrap together. Slice each wrap into 3 pieces, and serve.

TUMMY TAMER

To avoid added salt and preservatives, purchase a large turkey breast, roast it in the oven, and use it for salads, sandwiches, soups, pastas, and other dishes.

Roasted Pepper Hummus

Hummus is a savory dish that can be used as a creamy topping on various sandwiches or as a dip for fresh or steamed vegetables. This version is slightly sweet and perfectly creamy.

Yield:	**Prep time:**	**Serving size:**
1½ cups	10 minutes	2 tablespoons
Each serving has:		
107 calories	11 g carbohydrates	6 g fat
3 g fiber	4 g protein	

1 (15.5-oz.) can chickpeas, drained and rinsed

⅓ cup vegetable broth

¼ cup sesame tahini

¼ tsp. salt

¼ cup olive oil

1 cup roasted red peppers

1. In a blender, combine chickpeas, vegetable broth, sesame tahini, salt, olive oil, and roasted red peppers.
2. Purée until smooth. Serve with baby carrots and whole-wheat crackers.

Variation: You can substitute roasted eggplant or canned artichokes instead of the roasted red peppers for a great-tasting variation.

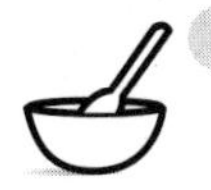

DEFINITION

Hummus is a thick, Middle Eastern spread made of puréed chickpeas (a.k.a. garbanzo beans), lemon juice, olive oil, garlic, and often tahini (sesame seed paste). In this recipe, lemon juice and garlic are omitted to keep you reflux free.

White Bean Artichoke Dip

Creamy and silky, this dip is savory and slightly salty and is a definite crowd pleaser.

Yield:	**Prep time:**	**Serving size:**
$2\frac{1}{2}$ cups	10 minutes	$\frac{1}{4}$ cup
Each serving has:		
95 calories	12 g carbohydrates	4 g fat
3 g fiber	4 g protein	

1 (15-oz.) can no-salt-added Great Northern beans, drained and rinsed

1 (13.75-oz.) can artichoke hearts, drained

$\frac{1}{4}$ cup fresh chopped cilantro

$\frac{1}{4}$ cup fresh chopped curly parsley

1 TB. olive oil

$\frac{1}{2}$ tsp. salt

1. In a blender, combine Great Northern beans, artichoke hearts, cilantro, parsley, olive oil, and salt.
2. Blend until smooth. Serve with vegetables, whole-wheat crackers, or baked tortilla chips.

TUMMY TAMER

This dip also goes well as a dressing on sandwiches or as a stand-alone sandwich spread.

Tzatziki Dip

Slightly sour, delightfully creamy, and with slight dill undertones, this dip pairs beautifully with the crunchiness of fresh cucumbers.

Yield:	**Prep time:**	**Serving size:**
2½ cups	10 minutes	2 tablespoons
Each serving has:		
21 calories	1 g carbohydrates	1 g fat
0 g fiber	2 g protein	

1 cup fat-free Greek yogurt

½ large cucumber, peeled, seeded, and julienned

1 TB. extra-virgin olive oil

2 TB. chopped fresh dill

2 TB. chopped fresh cilantro

¼ tsp. salt

1. In a small bowl, combine Greek yogurt, cucumber, extra-virgin olive oil, dill, cilantro, and salt.
2. Serve *tzatziki* with vegetables or as a sandwich topping.

DEFINITION

Tzatziki is a Greek dip traditionally made with Greek yogurt, cucumbers, garlic, and mint. Garlic and mint are omitted from this recipe to keep you reflux free.

Apple Chips

These sweet, zesty, and crunchy chips are perfect as a snack or mixed into plain fat-free yogurt.

Yield:	Prep time:	Cook time:	Serving size:
40 chips	5 minutes	$1\frac{1}{2}$ hours	20 chips
Each serving has:			
189 calories	25 g carbohydrates	4 g fat	5 g fiber
15 g protein			

2 medium Granny Smith apples, cored

2 tsp. confectioners' sugar

1 tsp. ground cinnamon

1. Preheat the oven to 200°F. Line a large baking sheet with parchment paper.
2. Cut apples into thin slices, and arrange in a single layer on the baking sheet. Sprinkle with confectioners' sugar and cinnamon.
3. Bake for about $1\frac{1}{2}$ hours or until apples begin to crisp. Remove from the oven and allow to cool before serving.

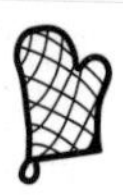

COOLER TALK

Cinnamon has many healthy properties such as stabilizing blood sugar levels and lowering LDL cholesterol levels. Sprinkle it liberally over your snacks, desserts, cereals, and baked goods.

Kale Chips

Slightly bitter, these kale chips are perfectly crunchy with just the right degree of cheesiness.

Yield:	**Prep time:**	**Cook time:**	**Serving size:**
6 cups	5 minutes	15 minutes	1 cup
Each serving has:			
47 calories	4 g carbohydrates	3 g fat	1 g fiber
2 g protein			

1 large head fresh kale

½ tsp. salt

1 TB. olive oil

2 TB. reduced-fat grated Parmesan cheese

1. Preheat the oven to 350°F.
2. Snip stems off kale leaves, and wash leaves under running water. Dry thoroughly with paper towels.
3. Using kitchen shears, snip kale into 1-inch pieces and place into a large bowl. Add salt, olive oil, and Parmesan cheese, tossing to coat.
4. Transfer onto a parchment paper–lined cookie sheet. Bake for 10 to 15 minutes. Kale should be crispy but not burned.

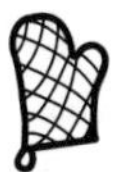

COOLER TALK

Kale has a long history. In the days of the Roman Empire, it used to be called sabelline cabbage. Today, it can help you get additional calcium into your diet. It's a great source of calcium and vitamins A, C, and E.

Potato Cakes

Potatoes are one of the best comfort foods out there, and these cheesy cakes covered with golden breadcrumbs really fit the bill. Better yet, make extras and freeze for later.

Yield:	**Prep time:**	**Cook time:**	**Serving size:**
10 cakes	20 minutes	10 minutes	2 cakes
Each serving has:			
154 calories	20 g carbohydrates	2 g fat	3 g fiber
13 g protein			

4 medium Yukon Gold potatoes

1 (6-oz.) can tuna, packed in water and drained

¼ cup fat-free shredded mozzarella cheese

¼ cup chopped fresh curly parsley

¼ cup chopped fresh dill

¼ tsp. salt

¼ cup whole-wheat breadcrumbs

1 TB. light butter

1. Place potatoes in a medium saucepan, cover with water, and set over high heat. Bring to a boil, lower heat to medium, and cook for about 20 to 25 minutes or until potatoes are fork-tender.
2. Pour out water, and mash potatoes. Add tuna, mozzarella cheese, parsley, dill, salt, and breadcrumbs.
3. In a large skillet over medium-high heat, heat light butter.
4. Form potato mixture into 10 (1-inch) patties, and add to the skillet. Cook for about 4 or 5 minutes per side or until golden brown. Serve warm.

TUMMY TAMER

Consider preparing this recipe, and many others, using cast-iron cookware. In addition to adding great flavor and extra iron to your food, cast-iron pans will last for generations. This will save lots of money on purchasing new cookware in the long run.

Majestic Surf Tapas

If you've never tried sardines, you may be surprised by this dish. Parsley and mayo, along with sage and other spices, take the "fishiness" out of these *tapas* and make this humble fish taste simply majestic.

Yield:	**Prep time:**	**Serving size:**
12 crackers	10 minutes	2 crackers
Each serving has:		
66 calories	2 g carbohydrates	4 g fat
0 g fiber	5 g protein	

2 large hard-boiled eggs, peeled and chopped

3 TB. canned corn

1 TB. grated Parmesan cheese

2 TB. light mayo

1 TB. chopped fresh parsley

$\frac{1}{4}$ tsp. sage powder

1 (3.75-oz.) can sardines, packed in water, drained, and finely chopped

$\frac{1}{8}$ tsp. salt

12 whole-wheat crackers

1. In a medium bowl, combine eggs, corn, Parmesan cheese, light mayo, parsley, and sage powder. Add sardines and salt and mix well.
2. Spread mixture evenly on the whole-wheat crackers, about 1 tablespoon per cracker.

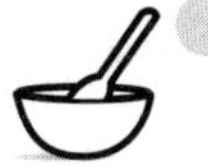

DEFINITION

Tapas is a Spanish term meaning "little plates" and collectively describes appetizers and snacks usually served as individual-size portions. Tapas can be either cold or warm.

Oven-Baked Cheese Sticks

Crunchy on the outside and warm and melted on the inside, these cheesy treats are a definite comfort food.

Yield:	Prep time:	Cook time:	Serving size:
8 cheese sticks	35 minutes	8 minutes	2 cheese sticks
Each serving has:			
283 calories	20 g carbohydrates	13 g fat	2 g fiber
19 g protein			

1 cup whole-wheat breadcrumbs
$\frac{1}{4}$ tsp. salt
$\frac{1}{2}$ tsp. dried oregano
$\frac{1}{4}$ tsp. dried basil
$\frac{1}{4}$ cup all-purpose flour
3 large egg whites, beaten
8 low-fat mozzarella cheese sticks

1. Line a cookie sheet with parchment paper.
2. In a medium bowl, combine breadcrumbs, salt, oregano, and basil. Set aside.
3. Pour flour into a shallow bowl.
4. Pour beaten egg whites into a separate shallow bowl.
5. Dip each mozzarella cheese stick in flour, in egg mixture, and in breadcrumbs, turning to coat. Transfer to the parchment paper–lined cookie sheet, and repeat with remaining sticks. Refrigerate for 30 minutes or up to 4 hours.
6. Preheat the oven to 400°F.
7. Bake for about 8 minutes. Serve warm.

TUMMY TAMER

Cheese sticks are a great way to get some bone-building calcium and muscle-building protein into your diet. The restaurant or freezer-case variety is loaded with calories and artery-clogging saturated fat. This recipe offers all the goodness without the unwanted impostors.

Scallop Spring Rolls

These treats are slightly crispy on the outside and perfectly seasoned and moist on the inside.

Yield:	**Prep time:**	**Cook time:**	**Serving size:**
6 rolls	15 minutes	15 minutes	2 rolls
Each serving has:			
272 calories 24 g protein	30 g carbohydrates	6 g fat	5 g fiber

1 TB. olive oil

6 button mushrooms, sliced

2 medium carrots, peeled and shredded

1 medium zucchini, julienned

1 tsp. salt

16 large scallops, quartered

6 rice paper wraps

Nonstick cooking spray

1. In a medium saucepan over medium-high heat, heat olive oil. When warm, add mushrooms, carrots, zucchini, and salt, and cook for about 5 minutes.
2. When vegetables begin to soften, add scallops and cook for 5 minutes or until scallops turn opaque and slightly brown. Remove from heat, and transfer to a separate dish.
3. Preheat the oven to 360°F. Lightly coat a baking sheet with nonstick cooking spray.
4. Dip each rice sheet individually into a bowl of cold water to soften. When soft, remove excess water with a paper towel.
5. Place about 3 heaping tablespoons of vegetable mixture in the center of each sheet, fold like an egg roll, and place on the prepared baking sheet. Lightly spray rolls with nonstick cooking spray. Bake for about 10 to 15 minutes or until rolls are slightly crispy and golden brown.

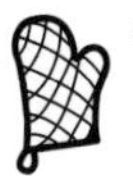

COOLER TALK

Scallops are also a good source of protein, which has been shown to help with acid reflux symptoms.

Sweet Popcorn

This is a perfect low-calorie alternative for soothing a sweet tooth. This crunchy popcorn is sweet and only takes minutes to make.

Yield: 4 cups	**Prep time:** 3 minutes	**Cook time:** 3 minutes	**Serving size:** 2 cups
Each serving has:			
94 calories	17 g carbohydrates	2 g fat	3 g fiber
3 g protein			

2 TB. plain popcorn kernels

1 TB. confectioners' sugar

1 TB. slivered almonds

$\frac{1}{4}$ tsp. ground cinnamon

1. Place plain popcorn in a brown lunch bag, and microwave on high for 2 or 3 minutes or until most kernels have popped.
2. Add confectioners' sugar, almonds, and ground cinnamon to the bag, and shake vigorously.
3. Transfer popcorn to a large serving platter, and enjoy warm.

Variation: For a savory version, spray hot popcorn with nonstick cooking spray and sprinkle with 2 tablespoons grated reduced-fat Parmesan cheese.

TUMMY TAMER

Low-fat homemade popcorn makes a great snack or a fun game-day appetizer. Movie theater versions, on the other hand, can be loaded with butter and extra calories that can add unwanted pounds and trigger acid reflux symptoms. Make your own version or stick with plain air-popped varieties instead.

Deviled Eggs

This recipe is slightly in between the traditional deviled eggs and tapenade-filled eggs, which incorporate olives into the recipe. These are an all-time party favorite treat.

Yield:	**Prep time:**	**Cook time:**	**Serving size:**
16 egg halves	10 minutes	30 minutes	2 egg halves
Each serving has:			
293 calories	4 g carbohydrates	21 g fat	1 g fiber
20 g protein			

- 8 hard-boiled eggs, peeled and sliced in half lengthwise
- ½ cup pitted and chopped large black olives
- ¼ tsp. salt
- ⅛ tsp. ground sage
- 3 TB. light canola mayonnaise

1. Scoop egg yolks from egg whites into a small bowl. Press yolks from 4 eggs through a sieve, and discard remaining 4 yolks.
2. Add egg yolks, black olives, salt, ground sage, and mayonnaise, and mix well.
3. Divide mixture among 16 egg white halves, and serve.

Variation: For variety of flavor and texture, consider adding 1 tablespoon canned tuna in water, drained, to the egg mixture when mixing. You may decorate with 1 parsley leaf on top of each egg.

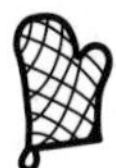

COOLER TALK

The color of the egg yolk comes from beta-carotene, a natural pigment found in plants that helps boost the immune system. Beta-carotene is also found in carrots.

Endive Cups with Avocado Salad

One bite of this salad, and your mouth explodes with multiple flavors and textures and leaves you craving more.

Yield: 12 endive cups	**Prep time:** 15 minutes	**Serving size:** 2 endive cups
Each serving has:		
144 calories	19 g carbohydrates	7 g fat
9 g fiber	5 g protein	

- 1 medium avocado, peeled, seeded, and chopped
- $^1/_2$ cup canned corn
- $^1/_4$ cup finely chopped celery
- $^1/_4$ tsp. salt
- $^1/_4$ cup chopped fresh cilantro
- 1 TB. chopped fresh parsley
- $^1/_4$ cup fat-free Greek yogurt
- 1 TB. 100 percent apple juice (not from concentrate)
- 1 medium head *endive*

1. In a small bowl, combine avocado, corn, celery, salt, cilantro, parsley, Greek yogurt, and apple juice.
2. Break endive leaves from their stems one by one. Wash thoroughly, and dry with paper towels.
3. Place endive leaves on a platter, and fill with equal portions of avocado mixture.

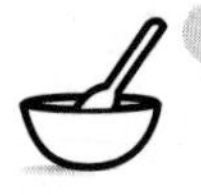

DEFINITION

Endive is a vegetable that resembles lettuce leaves but is slightly bitter tasting.

Stuffed Mushrooms

This classic cheesy party favorite will fill your mouth with amazing flavor.

Yield:	Prep time:	Cook time:	Serving size:
12 mushrooms	15 minutes	45 minutes	2 mushrooms
Each serving has:			
189 calories	25 g carbohydrates	4 g fat	5 g fiber
15 g protein			

2 TB. light butter

2 TB. all-purpose flour

1 cup fat-free milk

¼ tsp. salt

1 (10-oz.) pkg. frozen spinach, thawed

1 cup fat-free shredded mozzarella cheese

1 large egg, beaten

2 cups whole-wheat panko breadcrumbs

12 large white stuffer mushrooms

1. Preheat the oven to 375°F. Spray an 8×8-inch baking pan with nonstick cooking spray.
2. In a medium saucepan over medium-high heat, melt light butter and add all-purpose flour. Mix well, and cook for 30 to 60 seconds.
3. Slowly stir in fat-free milk and salt, and mix well to prevent clumping.
4. Squeeze out all liquid from thawed spinach, and add to the saucepan. Add mozzarella cheese, and mix well. Remove from heat, and set aside.
5. Pour egg into a small bowl.
6. Place breadcrumbs in a medium bowl.
7. Dip each mushroom into beaten egg and breadcrumbs, and add to the baking pan. Stuff each mushroom with 1 tablespoon spinach mixture.
8. Bake for about 35 minutes or until mushrooms are golden on the outside and soft on the inside.

Variation: If you like, you can substitute regular whole-wheat breadcrumbs instead.

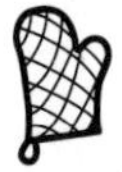

COOLER TALK

Whole-wheat panko breadcrumbs add unique flavor and texture to this dish as well as additional fiber.

Honey and Rosemary Flatbread

This flatbread is sweet and savory with just the right amount of herbed goodness.

Yield:	**Prep time:**	**Cook time:**	**Serving size:**
16 flatbreads	5 minutes	3 minutes	4 flatbreads
Each serving has:			
94 calories	15 g carbohydrates	4 g fat	1 g fiber
2 g protein			

1½ cups whole-wheat flour

1 tsp. baking powder

½ tsp. salt

½ cup water

¼ cup olive oil

¼ cup low-fat grated Parmesan cheese

⅓ cup honey

1 tsp. sea salt

1 TB. fresh rosemary, chopped

1. Preheat the oven to 450°F. Set a baking sheet on the middle rack.
2. In a medium bowl, whisk together whole-wheat flour, baking powder, and salt. Gradually add water and olive oil, and stir until dough forms. Knead dough gently several times on a work surface.
3. Split dough into 4 pieces. Roll out each piece on a sheet of parchment paper into a long cylindrical shape. Dough should be rolled thin and will feel oily.
4. Place dough and parchment paper onto the preheated baking sheet, and bake for about 5 minutes or until lightly golden brown. Remove from the oven and sprinkle each with ¼ of grated Parmesan cheese. Bake for 3 more minutes or until browned at edges.
5. Remove flatbreads from the oven. Immediately drizzle each with honey, sprinkle with sea salt, and garnish with rosemary. Cut each cracker widthwise into 4 sections. Serve warm.

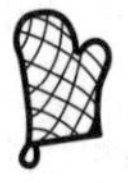

COOLER TALK

Rosemary is known for its antioxidant effects. In addition to bread, it pairs well with potatoes and many meat dishes.

Chapter 14

Super Soups and Sandwiches

In This Chapter

- Stomach-soothing broth-based soups
- Creamy soups to comfort your soul
- Decadent sandwiches to excite your taste buds

Soups aren't just a cold-weather treat. They're perfect year-round. In the wintertime, chicken noodle soups or creamy chowders warm you from the inside out. In the summertime, refreshing gazpachos provide soothing relief from the warm weather.

This chapter is filled with cold soups, warm soups, and accompanying sandwiches to create a complete meal for any time of the year. Just as with soups, sandwiches can be a creative mix of warm or cold, vegetarian or meat based, wrapped in whole-wheat tortillas or sandwiched between slices of juicy sourdough bread. Turn the page to introduce your taste buds to new and fun flavors!

Cold Coconut Thai-Infused Soup

This Thai-inspired soup blends the sweet flavors of coconut and corn with a little extra twist of cilantro.

Yield:	**Prep time:**	**Chill time:**	**Serving size:**
4 cups	5 minutes	1 hour or overnight	1 cup
Each serving has:			
255 calories	16 g carbohydrates	12 g fat	4 g fiber
5 g protein			

- $1\frac{1}{2}$ cups canned reduced-fat coconut milk
- 1 cup fat-free milk
- $\frac{1}{4}$ tsp. salt
- $\frac{1}{2}$ cup shelled edamame
- 1 medium avocado, peeled, seeded, and finely chopped
- 1 cup canned corn
- 1 TB. chopped fresh cilantro

1. In a blender, combine coconut milk, fat-free milk, salt, and edamame. Blend until smooth and transfer to a medium bowl.
2. Add avocado, corn, and cilantro, and mix well.
3. Chill for at least 1 hour or overnight. Serve in 4 individual bowls.

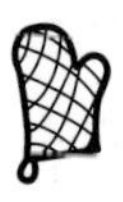

COOLER TALK

Avocado is not a vegetable but a fruit. It's a good source of healthy fats. But because even healthy fats can aggravate your acid reflux, keep your portion sizes under control and monitor your tolerance.

Chilled Cantaloupe Soup

This soup is sweet and smooth—ideal as an appetizer or a dessert.

Yield:	**Prep time:**	**Chill time:**	**Serving size:**
4 cups	10 minutes	1 to 4 hours	1 cup
Each serving has:			
86 calories	21 g carbohydrates	1 g fat	4 g fiber
2 g protein			

1 medium cantaloupe

1 TB. honey

¼ tsp. ground cinnamon

1 cup fresh blueberries

1 cup fresh blackberries

1. Slice cantaloupe in half, and scoop out the seeds. Peel off the rind, and roughly chop cantaloupe.
2. In a blender, combine cantaloupe, honey, and cinnamon. Blend until smooth.
3. Transfer to a large container, add blueberries and blackberries, and chill for 1 to 4 hours. Serve in 4 individual bowls.

Variation: This soup is extra tasty with 1 teaspoon slivered almonds sprinkled over the top prior to serving.

TUMMY TAMER

A regular blender works well with this recipe. However, a handheld blender may be a good investment. It takes up less space, is easier to clean, and makes the preparation of many recipes a cinch!

Ultimate Comfort Chicken Noodle Soup

This soup definitely equals comfort in a pot! Perfectly balanced with chunks of real chicken, it will leave your taste buds happy and your stomach satisfied.

Yield:	**Prep time:**	**Cook time:**	**Serving size:**
12 cups	15 minutes	25 minutes	1 cup
Each serving has:			
156 calories	14 g carbohydrates	7 g fat	1 g fiber
9 g protein			

6 cups low-sodium chicken broth

9 to 12 chicken tenders, diced into 1-in. pieces

1½ cups egg noodles

1½ cups shredded carrots

1 cup diced celery

6 medium bay leaves

½ tsp. salt

½ tsp. dried oregano

1. In a large pot over high heat, bring chicken broth to a boil. Add chicken tenders, egg noodles, carrots, celery, bay leaves, salt, and oregano, and return to a boil.
2. Reduce heat to low, cover, and cook for about 20 minutes or until all ingredients are cooked through. Remove bay leaves before serving warm in individual bowls.

TUMMY TAMER

Consider using whole-wheat egg noodles or pasta in this recipe for an added dose of dietary fiber, along with the vitamins and minerals that are generally lost in the conversion of the whole grain to the white flour. If you aren't keen on whole wheat, try using half whole-wheat noodles and half egg noodles until your taste buds adjust.

Creamy Potato and Corn Soup

This soup is so rich and creamy, no one would ever guess it's the lightest calorie and fat version of the old-time favorite comfort food you could make.

Yield:	**Prep time:**	**Cook time:**	**Serving size:**
12 cups	30 minutes	53 minutes	1 cup
Each serving has:			
129 calories	18 g carbohydrates	4 g fat	1 g fiber
6 g protein			

3 medium Yukon Gold potatoes, skin on and cubed

3 TB. light butter

3 TB. all-purpose flour

1 cup low-sodium chicken broth

$1\frac{1}{2}$ cups fat-free milk

$1\frac{1}{2}$ cups fat-free creamer

1 cup canned corn

1 cup fat-free shredded mozzarella cheese

1. Place potatoes in a large pot, cover with water, and set over high heat. Bring to a boil, and cook for about 15 to 20 minutes or until potatoes are fork-tender. Drain and set aside.
2. In a large saucepan over medium heat, melt light butter. Add flour, and cook, stirring frequently, for about 3 minutes.
3. Add potatoes, chicken broth, fat-free milk, fat-free creamer, and corn, and stir well to avoid clumping.
4. Add mozzarella cheese, reduce heat to low, and cook for 30 minutes, stirring every 5 to 10 minutes. Serve warm in individual bowls.

TUMMY TAMER

Don't peel your potatoes! The skin is full of fiber, vitamin C, and vitamin B_6. It also protects nutrients from escaping during the cooking process.

Pumpkin Soup

This soup is slightly sweet and savory at the same time. Its creaminess is comforting, and it goes well with a variety of other dishes.

Yield:	**Prep time:**	**Cook time:**	**Serving size:**
6 cups	5 minutes	30 minutes	$1\frac{1}{2}$ cups
Each serving has:			
195 calories	25 g carbohydrates	1 g fat	3 g fiber
20 g protein			

2 medium sweet potatoes, peeled and cut in half crosswise

1 cup unsweetened pumpkin purée

2 cups fat-free cream

$\frac{1}{4}$ tsp. ground cinnamon

$\frac{1}{8}$ tsp. ground ginger

$\frac{1}{8}$ tsp. salt

1. Place sweet potatoes in a medium saucepan, cover with water, and set over high heat. Bring to a boil, reduce heat to low, and cook for about 20 minutes or until sweet potatoes are fork-tender.
2. Pour out water, and add pumpkin purée and $1\frac{3}{4}$ cups cream to the saucepan. Add cinnamon, ginger, and salt, and return to a boil, stirring frequently.
3. Purée soup in batches in a blender, or using a handheld blender. Add remaining $\frac{1}{4}$ cup fat-free cream, and serve in 4 bowls.

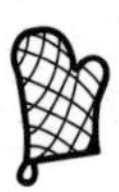

COOLER TALK

Pumpkin purée is generally sold in the baking aisle of the supermarket. Be sure to purchase 100 percent pumpkin purée and not the pumpkin pie filling, which often has sugar and flavoring added to it.

Melted Mozzarella and Fig Jam Sandwich

The aroma and flavor of the melted mozzarella cheese complement the sweetness of the fig jam in these surprising sandwiches.

Yield: 2 sandwiches	**Prep time:** 5 minutes	**Cook time:** 15 minutes	**Serving size:** 1 sandwich
Each serving has:			
162 calories	27 g carbohydrates	3 g fat	4 g fiber
9 g protein			

4 slices light whole-wheat bread (45 calories or less per slice)

2 TB. 100 percent natural fig jam

4 (1-oz.) slices reduced-fat mozzarella cheese

1. Preheat the oven to 425°F.
2. Place 2 (10×10-inch) pieces of aluminum foil on the countertop, and place 1 slice of bread in the middle of each piece of aluminum foil. Spread 1 tablespoon fig jam on each slice of bread, top each with 2 slices mozzarella cheese, and top with remaining bread slices. Wrap sandwiches in aluminum foil.
3. Bake for 10 minutes. Open the foil, and bake, uncovered, for another 5 minutes until cheese is melted and outside is slightly browned and crusty. Serve warm.

Variation: Many other jams go well with this recipe if you're not a fan of figs.

TUMMY TAMER

Many people use a panini press to make panini sandwiches. If you own one, feel free to utilize it in this recipe. If you don't have one, you can still make melted cheese sandwiches using your oven. Just be sure to preheat the oven first so the bread gets crispy on the outside while baking.

Hummus Avocado Sandwich

This vegetarian sandwich will please any palate—even a carnivore's!

Yield: 2 sandwiches	**Prep time:** 5 minutes	**Cook time:** 20 to 30 seconds	**Serving size:** 1 sandwich
Each serving has: 290 calories, 9 g protein	46 g carbohydrates	10 g fat	9 g fiber

2 medium whole-wheat pitas

4 TB. hummus

½ large avocado, peeled, seeded, and sliced into thin slices

¼ cup alfalfa sprouts

½ medium cucumber, peeled and seeded

1. Slice pitas around the top to form a pocket inside. Place on a plate, top with a slightly damp paper towel to prevent dehydration, and microwave on high for 20 to 30 seconds.
2. Fill each pita with 2 tablespoons hummus, ½ of avocado slices, ½ of alfalfa sprouts, and ½ of cucumber. Serve by itself or with a side of fruit, salad, or soup.

TUMMY TAMER

Extend the shelf life of bread products such as pitas and muffins by storing them in the refrigerator or freezing them for later use.

Falafel Pita Sandwich

This *falafel* wrap is perfectly juicy, flavorful, and moist.

Yield: 2 sandwiches	**Prep time:** 10 minutes	**Cook time:** 10 minutes	**Serving size:** 1 sandwich
Each serving has: 639 calories 22 g protein	100 g carbohydrates	19 g fat	17 g fiber

1 (15-oz.) can chickpeas, drained and rinsed
2 TB. all-purpose flour
2 TB. whole-wheat flour
1 TB. chopped fresh parsley leaves
1 TB. chopped fresh cilantro leaves
1 tsp. ground cumin
1 TB. apple juice
¼ tsp. salt
1 TB. walnut oil
2 medium whole-wheat pitas
2 TB. tahini paste
¼ cup cucumber, sliced thin
½ cup alfalfa sprouts

1. In a blender, purée chickpeas, all-purpose flour, whole-wheat flour, parsley, cilantro, cumin, apple juice, and salt.
2. Form mixture into 12 to 14 (1-inch) round patties.
3. In a large skillet over medium-high heat, heat walnut oil. When hot, add patties, and cook for about 3 minutes per side. Transfer cooked patties to a plate.
4. Add pitas to the skillet, warming for 1 minute on each side.
5. Place pitas on a plate, and slice around the top to form a pocket inside. Spread 1 tablespoon tahini paste inside each pita, top with cucumbers and alfalfa sprouts, and add an equal number of prepared patties. Serve warm.

DEFINITION

Falafel is a Middle Eastern food made of seasoned, ground chickpeas formed into patties or balls, cooked, and often used as a filling in pitas.

Baked Tuna "Panini"

This savory tuna sandwich features the flavors of melted cheese and fresh tarragon on slices of whole-wheat bread.

Yield:	**Prep time:**	**Cook time:**	**Serving size:**
2 sandwiches	10 minutes	15 minutes	1 sandwich
Each serving has:			
324 calories	33 g carbohydrates	7 g fat	5 g fiber
30 g protein			

1 (6-oz.) can tuna packed in water, drained

1/4 cup finely chopped celery

2 TB. light canola mayonnaise

2 TB. chopped fresh tarragon

1/4 tsp. salt

4 slices pumpernickel bread

1/4 cup fat-free shredded mozzarella cheese

1. Preheat the oven to 425°F.
2. In a small bowl, combine tuna, celery, light canola mayonnaise, tarragon, and salt.
3. Place 2 (10×10-inch) pieces of aluminum foil on the countertop, and place 1 slice of bread in the middle of each piece of aluminum foil. Top each piece of bread with 1/2 of tuna mixture. Top off with mozzarella cheese, and cover with remaining slices of bread. Wrap sandwiches in aluminum foil.
4. Bake for 10 minutes. Open the foil, and bake, uncovered, for 5 minutes. Serve warm.

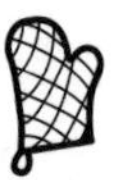

COOLER TALK

Tarragon is one of the ingredients in the traditional Dijon mustard recipe. It has bittersweet flavor and tastes slightly of licorice. In addition to mustard, it also goes well with fish, meat, and soups.

Chicken Pesto Sandwich

This sandwich combines three of the most popular ingredients—pesto, chicken, and cheese. Get ready for your new favorite sandwich!

Yield:	**Prep time:**	**Cook time:**	**Serving size:**
2 sandwiches	5 minutes	10 minutes	1 sandwich
Each serving has:			
464 calories	32 g carbohydrates	25 g fat	2 g fiber
26 g protein			

2 (4-oz.) boneless, skinless chicken breasts

¼ cup pesto sauce

2 slices reduced-fat Swiss cheese

½ cup Boston lettuce

4 (½-in.) slices sourdough bread, toasted

1. Spray a grill pan with nonstick cooking spray, and preheat to medium.
2. Place chicken breasts between two layers of plastic wrap, and pound until thin.
3. Add chicken breasts to the grill pan, and cook for 5 minutes or until golden brown. Flip over chicken, and cook other side for 5 minutes. When chicken is close to being done, spread ½ of pesto sauce on each chicken breast, and top with 1 slice Swiss cheese each.
4. Distribute Boston lettuce between 2 sourdough slices, place chicken on top, and top off with remaining 2 slices of bread. Serve as is or with a warm cup of soup.

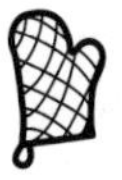

COOLER TALK

Traditional pesto is made with a mortar and pestle. To extract even more flavor, basil leaves are first crushed by hand.

Extraordinary Roast Beef Sandwich

In this sandwich, juicy roast beef combines with flavored cream cheese to provide an unforgettable combination.

Yield:	Prep time:	Serving size:
2 sandwiches	10 minutes	1 sandwich
Each serving has:		
286 calories	34 g carbohydrates	8 g fat
1 g fiber	21 g protein	

- $\frac{1}{4}$ cup whipped cream cheese
- $\frac{1}{2}$ tsp. chopped fresh dill
- $\frac{1}{4}$ tsp. chopped fresh parsley
- 2 (2-in.) baguettes, sliced open
- $\frac{1}{2}$ lb. cooked roast beef, thinly sliced

1. In a small bowl, combine whipped cream cheese with dill and parsley.
2. Top $\frac{1}{2}$ of each baguette with cream cheese mixture and $\frac{1}{2}$ of roast beef. Top with remaining bread, place on a plate, and serve by itself or with a cup of soup or salad.

TUMMY TAMER

Add more fiber to your sandwich by substituting medium whole-wheat wraps for the baguettes.

Apple Chicken Wrap

The juiciness of chicken pairs nicely with the sweetness and the crunchiness in this sweet and fresh wrap.

Yield:	**Prep time:**	**Serving size:**
4 wraps	15 minutes	1 wrap
Each serving has:		
489 calories	64 g carbohydrates	15 g fat
9 g fiber	26 g protein	

1 (16-oz.) can all-white chicken in water, drained

1 small Granny Smith apple, cored and finely chopped

¼ cup celery, finely chopped

¼ tsp. salt

¼ cup shredded carrots

⅓ cup light canola mayonnaise

4 TB. raisins

4 cups lettuce leaves

4 medium whole-wheat wraps

1. In a medium bowl, combine chicken, Granny Smith apple, celery, salt, carrots, light canola mayonnaise, and raisins. Mix well to coat.
2. Place 1 cup lettuce leaves on each whole-wheat wrap. Top with ¼ of chicken mixture. Fold and serve.

Variation: Change your turf to surf by substituting canned salmon for canned chicken.

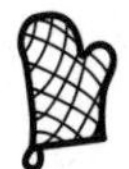

COOLER TALK

Contrary to a widely popular myth, celery is not a negative-calorie food. One cup chopped celery has 16 calories, 2 grams fiber, and 1 gram protein. This does, however, make celery a perfect low-calorie food to add volume without many extra calories.

Chapter 15

Sensational Salads

In This Chapter

- Fantastic salad dressings
- Seafood salads for all occasions
- Colorful vegetable crowd-pleasers

Salads are a fun and versatile way to add variety to any meal plan. For many acid reflux patients, they have been a big no-no because of the heavy and acidic dressings, not to mention the numerous acid reflux triggers such as bacon, croutons, and tomatoes. But no longer! This chapter is filled with recipes that will bring salads back into your life in a healthy and delicious way.

Creativity is the name of the game when it comes to salads. The recipes in this chapter take ordinary ingredients and combine them in many extraordinary ways to awaken your taste buds and get you excited about eating salads again.

Sesame Ginger Dressing

This spicy, sweet Asian-inspired dressing goes well with fish, meat, and vegetarian dishes.

Yield:	**Prep time:**	**Serving size:**
10 tablespoons	10 minutes	1 tablespoon
Each serving has:		
98 calories	3 g carbohydrates	10 g fat
0 g fiber	0 g protein	

- 3 TB. brown sugar
- 4 tsp. soy sauce
- 2 TB. toasted sesame oil
- $\frac{1}{3}$ cup vegetable oil
- 2 tsp. sesame seeds
- $\frac{1}{4}$ tsp. ground ginger

1. In a small bowl, combine brown sugar, soy sauce, toasted sesame oil, vegetable oil, sesame seeds, and ground ginger.
2. Refrigerate any unused salad dressing for later use.

TUMMY TAMER

Use a combination of black and white sesame seeds to add to the look of this dressing.

Honey Yogurt Dressing

This creamy, slightly sweet, and slightly tangy dressing is a great substitute for the traditional honey Dijon dressing.

Yield:	**Prep time:**	**Serving size:**
12 tablespoons	5 minutes	1 tablespoon
Each serving has:		
19 calories	3 g carbohydrates	1 g fat
0 g fiber	1 g protein	

½ cup fat-free Greek yogurt
¼ cup olive oil
2 TB. honey
1 tsp. ground ginger
¼ tsp. ground cumin

1. In a small bowl, combine Greek yogurt, olive oil, honey, ginger, and cumin.
2. Refrigerate any leftovers for later use.

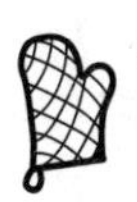

COOLER TALK

For every 1 pound honey, bees need to visit approximately 2 million flowers.

Seared Tuna Salad

This is a fun salad with many flavors and textures. Seaweed adds a savory crunch with a slightly chewy texture.

Yield:	**Prep time:**	**Cook time:**	**Serving size:**
2 cups	5 minutes	10 minutes (well done)	1 cup
Each serving has:			
570 calories	9 g carbohydrates	44 g fat	2 g fiber
33 g protein			

1 TB. sesame oil

2 TB. white sesame seeds

2 TB. black sesame seeds

1 (4-oz.) tuna steak

½ cup spinach leaves

½ cup arugula leaves

1 TB. Sesame Ginger Dressing (recipe earlier in this chapter)

¼ cup seaweed salad

1. In a small skillet over high heat, heat sesame oil.
2. On a small plate, combine white sesame seeds and black sesame seeds. Press both sides of tuna steak into sesame seeds to coat.
3. Add tuna to the skillet, and cook for 2 or 3 minutes per side or until golden brown. (If you like your fish well done, reduce heat to medium-low, cover the skillet, and cook for a few minutes longer until tuna is well done and no longer pink inside.)
4. Meanwhile, in a small bowl, toss spinach and arugula leaves, and add Sesame Ginger Dressing.
5. Arrange greens on a plate, and top with seaweed salad. Place warm tuna steak on top of greens, and serve.

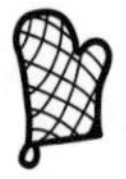

COOLER TALK

Seaweed can only survive in salt water. The rubbery exterior of the seaweed allows it to control the amount of salt it absorbs.

Shrimp and Cucumber Salad

This salad has a slight flavor of cilantro, which pairs nicely with the taste and texture of the shrimp.

Yield:	**Prep time:**	**Serving size:**
10 cups	10 minutes	5 cups
Each serving has:		
127 calories	14 g carbohydrates	2 g fat
3 g fiber	16 g protein	

4 TB. fat-free plain yogurt

2 TB. 100 percent apple juice (not from concentrate)

¼ tsp. salt

16 large cooked shrimp, shells and tails removed

1 large cucumber, thinly sliced

8 cups mixed greens, chopped

¼ cup chopped fresh dill

¼ cup chopped fresh cilantro

1. In a large bowl, combine yogurt, apple juice, and salt.
2. Add shrimp, cucumber, mixed greens, dill, and cilantro, and mix well to coat.

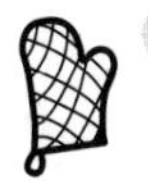

COOLER TALK

Shrimp is a great source of lean protein. Shrimp's high cholesterol content might be a concern for some people, so be sure to diversify your protein sources.

Jicama Salad

This salad tastes like spring on your plate, thanks to the crunch of fresh celery and *jicama*, and the sweetness of carrots, raisins, and apple juice.

Yield:	**Prep time:**	**Serving size:**
1 salad	10 minutes	$\frac{1}{2}$ of salad
Each serving has:		
261 calories	49 g carbohydrates	7 g fat
0 g fiber	4 g protein	

2 cups shredded carrot

2 cups peeled and julienned jicama

$\frac{1}{2}$ cup diced celery

$\frac{1}{4}$ cup raisins

$\frac{1}{4}$ tsp. salt

2 TB. 100 percent apple juice (not from concentrate)

1 TB. olive oil

1. In a medium bowl, combine carrot, jicama, celery, raisins, salt, apple juice, and olive oil.
2. Mix well, and serve.

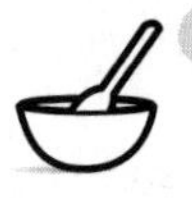

DEFINITION

Jicama is a juicy, crunchy, sweet, large, round Central American vegetable that's eaten both raw and cooked. It's available in many large grocery stores as well as from specialty vendors. If you can't find jicama, try substituting sliced water chestnuts.

Artichoke Rice Salad

In this creamy and filling salad, the chewiness of the brown rice complements the saltiness and the texture of black olives and canned artichokes.

Yield:	**Prep time:**	**Serving size:**
3 cups	10 minutes	1 cup
Each serving has:		
321 calories	45 g carbohydrates	14 g fat
11 g fiber	6 g protein	

2 cups cooked brown rice

1 (14-oz.) can artichoke hearts in water, drained

1 cup chopped black olives

1 tsp. salt

⅓ cup light canola mayonnaise

1. In a large bowl, combine brown rice, artichoke hearts, black olives, salt, and light canola mayonnaise.
2. Serve in 3 bowls.

TUMMY TAMER

The current recommendation for sodium is 1,500 milligrams per day, which translates into a little more than ½ teaspoon added salt. The recipes in this book use the minimal amount of salt for flavor, but you can skip it altogether or use less if you desire.

Russian Potato Salad

This is the Eastern European version of the American classic comfort food. The taste and flavor combinations of this recipe are very similar to the classic potato salad.

Yield:	**Prep time:**	**Cook time:**	**Serving size:**
6 cups	10 minutes	20 to 25 minutes	1 cup
Each serving has:			
333 calories	28 g carbohydrates	13 g fat	4 g fiber
25 g protein			

- 1½ lb. fingerling red potatoes
- 1 (15-oz.) can baby peas, drained
- 5 large hard-boiled eggs, peeled and chopped
- 2 cups finely chopped chicken breast
- ½ cup cucumber, peeled, seeded, and finely chopped
- ½ tsp. salt
- ½ tsp. dried dill weed
- ½ cup light canola mayonnaise

1. Place potatoes in a large pot, cover with water, and set over high heat. Bring to a boil, reduce heat to low, and simmer for 20 to 25 minutes or until potatoes are fork-tender.
2. Drain off water, and allow potatoes to cool slightly.
3. Cut potatoes into ¼-inch pieces, and place in a large bowl.
4. Add peas, eggs, chicken, cucumber, salt, dill weed, and light canola mayonnaise, and mix well. Serve warm or refrigerate for later.

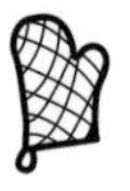

COOLER TALK

The first documentation of the potato was in 400 C.E., near the Lake Titicaca region between Peru and Bolivia.

Middle Eastern Cold Salad

This salad has both sweet and savory undertones paired with the delicious crunchiness of nuts.

Yield:	**Prep time:**	**Serving size:**
5 cups	10 minutes	1 cup
Each serving has:		
410 calories	78 g carbohydrates	6 g fat
10 g fiber	15 g protein	

1½ cups cooked couscous

1 (15-oz.) can chickpeas, drained and rinsed

¼ cup shredded carrots

½ tsp. ground cumin

¼ tsp. salt

½ cup golden raisins

¼ cup chopped fresh parsley

¼ cup chopped fresh cilantro

1 TB. extra-virgin olive oil

1. In a large bowl, combine couscous, chickpeas, carrots, cumin, salt, raisins, parsley, cilantro, and extra-virgin olive oil.
2. Serve in individual bowls.

TUMMY TAMER

Cumin is a rich source of fiber, iron, copper, calcium, and antioxidants. Use it to flavor soups and season meats.

Waldorf Carrot Salad

The original Waldorf salad was first presented at the world-famous Astoria hotel in 1893. This is my twist, made with carrots and raisins—sweet, crunchy, and juicy.

Yield:	**Prep time:**	**Chill time:**	**Serving size:**
8 cups	15 minutes	15 to 30 minutes	2 cups
Each serving has:			
223 calories	42 g carbohydrates	5 g fat	8 g fiber
7 g protein			

6 cups shredded carrots

1 medium Granny Smith apple, cored and finely chopped

½ cup raisins

¼ cup diced celery

¼ cup finely chopped raw walnuts

⅛ tsp. salt

½ cup fat-free Greek yogurt

3 TB. 100 percent apple juice (not from concentrate)

1. In a large bowl, combine carrots, Granny Smith apple, raisins, celery, walnuts, salt, Greek yogurt, and apple juice.
2. Chill for 15 to 30 minutes before serving to allow flavors to meld.

TUMMY TAMER

One celery stalk is about 10 calories. High volume and low calorie count makes celery a perfect mid-afternoon snack.

Beet, Goat Cheese, and Walnut Salad

This salad combines the sweetness of the beets with the creaminess of goat cheese and the crunchiness of walnuts for a mouthwatering creation that will have you asking for seconds.

Yield:	**Prep time:**	**Serving size:**
5 cups	10 minutes	2½ cups
Each serving has:		
198 calories	15 g carbohydrates	12 g fat
4 g fiber	10 g protein	

8 small baby beets, cooked, peeled, and chopped into ¼-in. pieces (about 1½ cups)

2 cups raw spinach

¼ tsp. salt

¼ cup goat cheese, crumbled

2 TB. 100 percent apple juice (not from concentrate)

¼ cup fat-free Greek yogurt

¼ cup finely chopped walnuts

1. In a medium bowl, combine beets, spinach, salt, goat cheese, apple juice, Greek yogurt, and walnuts.
2. Serve in 2 bowls.

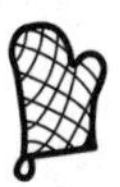

COOLER TALK

Goat cheese is naturally lower in saturated fat than many of the cow cheese varieties. It's a good alternative when you're craving the richness of cheese without extra fat and calories.

Zucchini and Almond Pasta Salad

This recipe is savory, rich, and crunchy due to the added slivered almonds.

Yield:	**Prep time:**	**Cook time:**	**Serving size:**
8 cups	10 minutes, plus overnight refrigeration	15 minutes	2 cups
Each serving has:			
275 calories	36 g carbohydrates	11 g fat	6 g fiber
13 g protein			

2/3 cup fat-free buttermilk

1/4 cup low-fat mayonnaise

2 TB. fresh parsley, minced

1/2 lb. whole-wheat rotini pasta

2 cups haricot verts

1/2 cup slivered almonds

2 medium zucchinis, thinly sliced lengthwise

1/2 cup low-fat Parmesan cheese, freshly shaved

1/8 tsp. salt

1. In a small bowl, combine buttermilk, mayonnaise, and parsley. Cover and refrigerate overnight.
2. Fill a large saucepan with 3 quarts water, set over high heat, and bring to a boil. Add whole-wheat rotini, and cook for about 7 minutes, stirring frequently, until rotini is tender. Drain, transfer rotini to a large wide bowl, and toss until cooled slightly. Set aside to cool completely.
3. Fill the large saucepan with 4 cups water, return to high heat, and bring to a boil. Add haricot verts, and cook for about 5 minutes. Drain haricot verts and run under cold water for about 30 seconds. Set aside to cool completely.
4. Preheat the oven to 350°F.
5. Toast slivered almonds on a small, nonstick baking tray for about 5 minutes or until golden brown. Set aside.
6. In a large bowl, toss rotini with zucchini, Parmesan cheese, and enough buttermilk dressing to coat. Top with slivered almonds, season with salt, and serve cold.

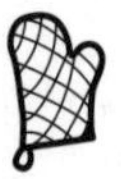

COOLER TALK

Haricot verts are also called French beans. They're crunchy and sweet, low in calories, and a good source of fiber. Add them to your salads, serve them as a side dish, or simply enjoy them as a snack.

Couscous Salad

This crunchy, salty, and savory salad has a delightful texture and flavor, thanks to the cheese and olives.

Yield:	**Prep time:**	**Cook time:**	**Serving size:**
1 salad	10 minutes, plus 1 hour chill time	5 minutes	¼ of salad
Each serving has:			
359 calories	48 g carbohydrates	12 g fat	3 g fiber
15 g protein			

1½ cups couscous
1¼ cups chicken broth
2 TB. olive oil
½ cup low-fat feta cheese
10 chopped black olives
⅓ cup chopped fresh parsley
2 TB. pine nuts

1. Place couscous in a medium bowl, and set aside.
2. In a small saucepan over high heat, bring chicken broth to a boil. Pour over couscous, and set aside for about 5 minutes or until all liquid is absorbed.
3. Add olive oil, feta cheese, black olives, parsley, and pine nuts, and mix to combine.
4. Refrigerate for 1 to 4 hours prior to serving.

ACID ALERT

Fiber has been shown to help reduce acid reflux symptoms. For added fiber in this recipe, consider using whole-wheat couscous.

Surf and Turf Entrées

Chapter 16

In This Chapter

- Meat-based comfort foods
- Sizzling steak recipes
- Fish for every palate

If you're a steak-and-potatoes kind of eater, this chapter is perfect for you. Enjoy your fish? There are plenty of recipes for you as well! From succulent meatballs to rosemary-flavored scallops, these dishes will awaken your taste buds and leave your stomach full and happy.

The recipes in this chapter are so easy to prepare that they're ideal for both novice cooks and expert chefs alike. Healthy, restaurant-inspired meals that take a short time to prepare are about to become a reality. Have fun cooking and eating!

Filet Mignon with Creamy Mushroom Sauce

Juicy, creamy, and flavorful—this dish is bound to make your mouth water.

Yield:	**Prep time:**	**Cook time:**	**Serving size:**
4 filets	15 minutes	15 minutes	1 filet
Each serving has:			
438 calories	10 g carbohydrates	29 g fat	1 g fiber
34 g protein			

5 TB. light butter

1 cup diced shiitake mushrooms

¼ cup diced portobello mushrooms

¼ tsp. salt

2 TB. all-purpose flour

½ cup low-sodium chicken broth

1 cup fat-free cream

4 (4-oz.) beef tenderloin filets, 1½-in. thick

1. In a medium saucepan over medium-high heat, melt 3 tablespoons light butter. Add shiitake mushrooms, portobello mushrooms, and salt, and cook for about 5 minutes or until golden brown.
2. Add flour, and mix thoroughly with a spoon or spatula.
3. Slowly add chicken broth, stirring to avoid clumps. Add fat-free cream, stirring to avoid clumps. Continue stirring as mixture heats. Remove from heat as soon as sauce starts gently boiling and is slightly thickened.
4. In a medium skillet over medium-high heat, melt remaining 2 tablespoons light butter. Add beef filets, and cook for about 5 to 7 minutes per side. For well-done steak, reduce heat to medium, cover, and cook for 5 to 10 minutes longer or until beef is nicely browned on both sides but not overcooked.
5. Serve each filet topped with ¼ of mushroom sauce.

TUMMY TAMER

For a lower-fat substitute, try bison filet mignon instead of beef. On average, bison meat is 25 percent leaner than beef.

Baked Meatballs

These meatballs are flavorful and juicy. The hardest part isn't making them, but stopping at one serving!

Yield:	**Prep time:**	**Cook time:**	**Serving size:**
9 meatballs	30 minutes	18 minutes	3 meatballs
Each serving has:			
478 calories	11 g carbohydrates	23 g fat	0 g fiber
56 g protein			

1 lb. 90 percent lean ground beef
¼ cup chopped fresh parsley
½ tsp. salt
¼ cup whole-wheat breadcrumbs
1 large egg
1 large egg white
¼ cup old-fashioned oats
2 TB. grated Parmesan cheese
½ cup fat-free shredded mozzarella cheese
1 tsp. dried oregano

1. Preheat the oven to 350°F. Spray a baking sheet with nonstick cooking spray.
2. In a large bowl, combine ground beef, parsley, salt, breadcrumbs, egg, egg white, oats, Parmesan cheese, mozzarella cheese, and oregano. Form mixture into 9 small (2-tablespoon) meatballs.
3. Place meatballs on the prepared baking sheet, and bake for 18 minutes or until no pink areas remain.

TUMMY TAMER

Meatballs are a versatile and fun dish. Serve them with lasagna, make meatball subs, or pair them with a side of healthy mashed cauliflower.

Mini Shepherd's Pies

Moist and flavorful on the inside and creamy on the outside, these little comfort creations are perfectly portioned to satisfy your craving.

Yield:	**Prep time:**	**Cook time:**	**Serving size:**
6 pies	25 minutes	25 minutes	1 pie
Each serving has:			
243 calories	20 g carbohydrates	9 g fat	3 g fiber
21 g protein			

3 medium Yukon Gold potatoes
2 TB. fat-free Greek yogurt
4 TB. light butter
¼ cup skim milk
¼ tsp. salt
1 cup mixed frozen vegetables
2 TB. all-purpose flour
¾ cup fat-free cream
½ cup low-sodium chicken broth
½ lb. 90 percent lean ground beef
¼ cup fat-free shredded mozzarella cheese

1. Place potatoes in a medium saucepan, cover with water, and set over high heat. Bring to a boil, reduce heat to medium, and cook for about 20 to 25 minutes or until potatoes are fork-tender.
2. Pour out liquid. Add Greek yogurt, 1 tablespoon light butter, skim milk, and ⅛ teaspoon salt, and mash well.
3. Preheat the oven to 425°F. Spray 6 (6-oz.) ramekins with nonstick cooking spray.
4. In a large skillet over medium-high heat, melt remaining 3 tablespoons light butter. Add frozen vegetables, and cook for about 5 to 7 minutes or until vegetables are thawed and slightly browned.
5. Add flour, and mix to coat. Slowly add fat-free cream, stirring to avoid clumps. Add chicken broth, stirring to prevent clumps.
6. Add remaining ⅛ teaspoon salt and beef. Mix well, using a spatula to break up any clumps. Add mozzarella cheese, mix well, and remove from heat.
7. Divide meat mixture evenly among ramekins, and top with mashed potatoes. Place the ramekins on a cookie sheet, and bake for 25 minutes or until tops are golden brown.

Mini Rosemary Souvlaki

The combination of rosemary and olive oil along with the sweetness of honey bring out the juicy flavors of the tender sirloin steak tips.

Yield:	**Prep time:**	**Cook time:**	**Serving size:**
8 skewers	10 minutes, plus 2 or 3 hours marinate time	15 minutes	2 skewers
Each serving has:			
260 calories 26 g protein	18 g carbohydrates	10 g fat	0 g fiber

¼ cup honey

2 TB. olive oil

1 TB. dried rosemary

½ tsp. salt

1 lb. sirloin tip steaks

1. In a small bowl, whisk together honey, olive oil, rosemary, and salt. Pour marinade into a zipper-lock plastic bag, add steak, seal, and toss to coat. Refrigerate for 2 or 3 hours.
2. Preheat the grill to medium-high. Lightly oil the grill rack or grill pan.
3. Remove steak from marinade, and discard marinade. Cut steak into 8 strips and thread onto 8 skewers.
4. Cook for 10 to 15 minutes, turning skewers frequently to ensure equal cooking.

ACID ALERT

Many restaurant souvlaki recipes have added garlic and other reflux-triggering ingredients. Make your own and keep your taste buds *and* your stomach happy!

Stuffed Flank Steak

This dish is moist and juicy with a perfect combination of spice, sweetness, and savory. Every bite of this steak is a sublime experience.

Yield:	**Prep time:**	**Cook time:**	**Serving size:**
1 steak	15 minutes	30 minutes	$\frac{1}{6}$ steak
Each serving has:			
408 calories	11 g carbohydrates	15 g fat	1 g fiber
56 g protein			

2 lb. flank steak

1 TB. dried rosemary

$\frac{1}{4}$ tsp. salt

3 cups baby spinach

$\frac{1}{2}$ cup raisins

$\frac{1}{4}$ cup fat-free shredded mozzarella cheese

1. Preheat the oven to 375°F.
2. *Butterfly* flank steak, and season on the inside with rosemary and salt.
3. Lay steak flat in a baking dish, and layer spinach, raisins, and mozzarella cheese on top. Roll steak over filling, using toothpicks to hold meat in place.
4. Bake for 30 minutes or until steak is done to the desired level of readiness.

Variation: For flavor variety, consider using an equal amount of sautéed broccoli rabe instead of spinach in this recipe.

DEFINITION

Butterfly means to slice a cut of meat in the middle without cutting all the way through. When you fold it open, it looks like a butterfly. Cut flank steak across the grain for maximum softness and pleasant chewing.

Veal Cutlets

This dish has a crunch on the outside and tenderness on the inside with a refreshing addition of fresh parsley.

Yield:	**Prep time:**	**Cook time:**	**Serving size:**
4 cutlets	10 minutes	25 minutes	2 cutlets
Each serving has:			
240 calories	15 g carbohydrates	12 g fat	3 g fiber
57 g protein			

2 cups whole-wheat breadcrumbs
$\frac{1}{2}$ cup chopped fresh curly parsley
5 TB. grated Parmesan cheese
4 medium egg whites
$\frac{1}{2}$ lb. *veal* cutlets (4 total)

1. Preheat the oven to 375°F. Line a baking sheet with parchment paper.
2. In a small bowl, combine breadcrumbs, parsley, and Parmesan cheese.
3. Pour egg whites in a small bowl.
4. Dip veal cutlets into egg whites and then into breadcrumb mixture to coat. Arrange cutlets on the prepared baking sheet.
5. Bake for 20 to 25 minutes or until golden brown on the outside and baked through on the inside.

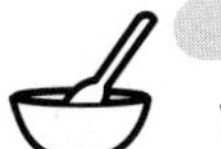

DEFINITION

Veal is meat from a calf, generally characterized by mild flavor and tenderness. Certain cuts of veal, such as cutlets and scaloppini, are well suited to quick cooking.

Root Vegetable Lamb Stew

This comfort-food stew is tender and melts in your mouth. It'll leave you satisfied and happy.

Yield:	**Prep time:**	**Cook time:**	**Serving size:**
8 cups	25 minutes	1 hour, 6 minutes	1 cup
Each serving has:			
390 calories	28 g carbohydrates	12 g fat	4 g fiber
41 g protein			

2 TB. light butter

2 lb. lamb stew meat, cubed

2 TB. all-purpose flour

2 cups vegetable broth

3 cups peeled and chopped rutabaga

1 cup peeled and chopped turnips

2 cups peeled and chopped eggplant

$1\frac{1}{2}$ cups Yukon Gold potatoes, skin on and diced

$1\frac{1}{2}$ cups *yucca root,* peeled and diced

1 cup parsnip, peeled and diced

6 bay leaves

1 tsp. salt

1 tsp. ground ginger

1. In a large pot over medium-high heat, melt light butter. Add stew meat, and cook for about 2 to 4 minutes or until golden brown on all sides.
2. Add flour, and cook for 2 minutes. Slowly add vegetable broth, stirring to avoid clumps.
3. Add rutabaga, turnips, eggplant, potatoes, yucca root, parsnip, bay leaves, salt, and ginger. Bring to a gentle boil, reduce heat to low, cover, and cook for 1 hour.
4. Turn off heat, and allow stew to rest for a few minutes before removing bay leaves and serving.

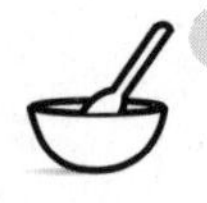

DEFINITION

Yucca root is a woody shrub with a root that's firm and tapered and resembles the shape of a sweet potato. It has a bittersweet flavor.

Pork Medallions with Fennel

Fennel adds a slightly sweet yet savory flavor to this tender pork dish.

Yield:	**Prep time:**	**Cook time:**	**Serving size:**
16 pieces	10 minutes	10 minutes	2 pieces
Each serving has:			
210 calories	3 g carbohydrates	5 g fat	1 g fiber
36 g protein			

3 lb. pork tenderloin, cut into 1-in.-thick medallions

1 tsp. salt

$\frac{1}{2}$ tsp. chopped fresh rosemary

$\frac{1}{2}$ tsp. fresh thyme, chopped

1 tsp. olive oil

1 fennel bulb, sliced

1 cup low-sodium chicken broth

1. Season pork medallions with salt, rosemary, and thyme.
2. In a large saucepan over medium-high heat, heat olive oil. Add pork medallions, and brown for about 2 minutes per side or until fully cooked.
3. Add fennel, reduce heat to medium, and add chicken broth. Cover and cook for 5 to 10 minutes or until fennel is translucent and pork is cooked through.

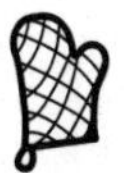

COOLER TALK

The Mediterranean is the homeland of fennel. Fennel is often confused for celery.

Salmon Burgers

These juicy burgers are perfect plain or used as a topping for salads or sandwiches.

Yield:	Prep time:	Cook time:	Serving size:
4 burgers	15 minutes	10 minutes	1 burger
Each serving has:			
345 calories	10 g carbohydrates	20 g fat	1 g fiber
32 g protein			

1 TB. light butter

2 cups loosely packed canned salmon, drained

$1\frac{1}{2}$ cups canned corn

$\frac{1}{4}$ cup all-purpose flour

$\frac{1}{4}$ cup whole-wheat breadcrumbs

$\frac{1}{2}$ cup fresh chopped parsley

$\frac{1}{4}$ tsp. salt

1. In a large skillet over medium-high heat, heat light butter.
2. In a large bowl, combine salmon, corn, flour, breadcrumbs, parsley, and salt. Form mixture into 4 patties.
3. Add patties to the skillet, and cook for about 5 minutes per side or until golden brown and cooked through on the inside.
4. Serve alone on the plate, on top of a salad, or inside toasted burger buns.

TUMMY TAMER

For a special occasion, use fresh ground salmon instead of the canned counterpart.

Poached Salmon with Yogurt Dressing

The tender salmon in this recipe pairs nicely with the creamy yogurt dressing flavored with dill and fennel.

Yield:	**Prep time:**	**Cook time:**	**Serving size:**
4 fillets	10 minutes	15 minutes	1 fillet
Each serving has:			
286 calories	4 g carbohydrates	16 g fat	1 g fiber
31 g protein			

4 cups low-sodium chicken broth

¼ tsp. salt

3 medium bay leaves

4 (4-oz.) salmon fillets, with skin

1 cup fat-free Greek yogurt

¼ cup fresh chopped fennel weed

¼ cup fresh chopped dill

1. In a large, deep skillet over medium-high heat, bring chicken broth to a boil. Add ⅛ teaspoon salt and bay leaves. Add salmon fillets, skin side down, and cook for about 5 to 7 minutes or to the desired degree of readiness. (If salmon is not completely covered by liquid, flip over once during cooking to ensure salmon is cooked all the way through.)
2. Meanwhile, in a small bowl, combine Greek yogurt, remaining ⅛ teaspoon salt, fennel, and dill.
3. Using a spatula, remove salmon to 4 plates, being careful to leave bay leaves in the pan. Distribute yogurt sauce equally over top before serving.

TUMMY TAMER

Salmon is a preferred item when it comes to getting omega-3 fatty acids in your diet. It's recommended that you consume fish at least twice a week for optimal health benefits.

Pesto-Crusted Tilapia

Pesto gives this dish an unbelievable aroma and flavor, and the cheesiness of the pesto and the flavor of basil go well with the texture and flavor of the whitefish.

Yield:	**Prep time:**	**Cook time:**	**Serving size:**
2 fillets	10 minutes	4 minutes	1 fillet
Each serving has:			
123 calories	2 g carbohydrates	5 g fat	0 g fiber
18 g protein			

2 (3-oz.) tilapia fillets

⅛ tsp. salt

4 tsp. pesto sauce

1. Spray a medium skillet with nonstick cooking spray, and set over medium-high heat.
2. Rub tilapia fillets with equal amounts of salt and pesto sauce, and add to the skillet. Cook for 2 minutes per side.

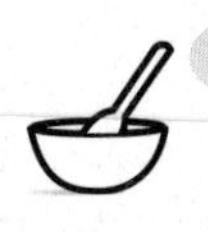

DEFINITION

Pesto is a thick spread or sauce made with fresh basil leaves, garlic, olive oil, pine nuts, and Parmesan cheese. Some newer versions are made with other herbs. You can make pesto at home or purchase it in a grocery store. It's tasty on anything from appetizers to pasta and other main dishes.

Peanut Sesame–Marinated Salmon

The combination of peanut and sesame oils along with the other ingredients add pleasant Asian-inspired flavor to this recipe.

Yield:	Prep time:	Cook time:	Serving size:
4 fillets	10 minutes, plus 4 hours or overnight marinate time	10 minutes	1 fillet
Each serving has:			
487 calories	3 g carbohydrates	36 g fat	0 g fiber
35 g protein			

¼ tsp. salt
¼ tsp. ground ginger
¼ cup toasted sesame oil
¼ cup peanut oil
3 TB. low-sodium soy sauce
2 tsp. brown sugar
4 (6-oz.) salmon fillets

1. In a medium bowl, combine salt, ginger, toasted sesame oil, peanut oil, soy sauce, and brown sugar.
2. Add salmon fillets, and marinate for 4 hours or overnight.
3. In a medium skillet over medium-high heat, cook salmon fillets for about 5 minutes per side or until desired readiness. Serve with a side salad, mashed potatoes, pasta, or alone.

TUMMY TAMER

Not a big fan of fish? This dish may be ideal for you. The marinade adds an intense flavor and aroma that covers the fish flavor, which may just make you reconsider salmon in the future.

Cod En Papillote

As soon as you rip open the parchment paper enclosing this dish, the room will fill with flavor and aroma. As a bonus, no additional calories and fat are added.

Yield:	Prep time:	Cook time:	Serving size:
4 fillets	10 minutes	20 minutes	1 fillet
Each serving has:			
109 calories	3 g carbohydrates	1 g fat	1 g fiber
22 g protein			

4 (4-oz.) cod fillets

½ tsp. salt

1 TB. low-sodium soy sauce

2 tsp. ground ginger

16 asparagus spears, tough ends snapped off

1. Preheat the oven to 400°F.
2. Place 4 (10×10-inch) pieces of parchment paper on the countertop. Place 1 cod fillet in the middle of each piece of parchment paper. Rub equal amounts of salt on each fillet, and cover with soy sauce and ginger. Arrange 4 asparagus spears on each fillet.
3. Tightly wrap the parchment paper around filling, transfer to a cookie sheet, and bake for 15 minutes.
4. Unwrap, transfer to a plate, and enjoy.

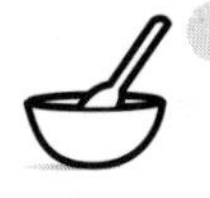

DEFINITION

En papillote is a cooking method wherein the food is placed in a folded pouch, normally parchment-type paper. The pouch is tightly sealed to create a closed environment that will help steam the food while preserving the flavor.

Rosemary Scallops

Aromatic rosemary brings out the flavor of juicy and meaty scallops.

Yield: 8 scallops	**Prep time:** 5 minutes	**Cook time:** 10 minutes	**Serving size:** 4 scallops
Each serving has:			
268 calories	9 g carbohydrates	7 g fat	0 g fiber
39 g protein			

2 TB. light butter
8 large scallops
1 TB. all-purpose flour
2 TB. chopped fresh rosemary
$\frac{1}{4}$ tsp. salt

1. In a medium skillet over medium-high heat, heat light butter.
2. Toss scallops in flour, and add to the skillet. Add rosemary and salt. Cook for about 2 to 4 minutes per side or until golden brown and cooked through.

TUMMY TAMER

Scallops are a fantastic source of protein, magnesium, phosphorous, potassium, selenium, and vitamin B_{12}. They're also very low in saturated fat.

Chapter 17

Poultry Pleasers

In This Chapter

- Turkey loafs and burgers
- Mouthwatering, lean comfort recipes
- Tasty marinated chicken creations

Poultry is a great way to add protein to your diet and can be prepared in many versatile ways. The Turkey Meatloaf that kicks off this chapter is just as moist and flavorful as an old-fashioned meatloaf. And turkey burgers make a great weekday dinner or can be prepared as a treat for a summer barbecue. The chicken recipes that follow include stuffed breasts, marinades, and skewers.

The recipes in this chapter are low in fat, high in protein, and packed with flavor. They're a great way to introduce your family to healthy eating.

Turkey Meatloaf

This loaf is colored with bright vegetables and tastes moist and delicious.

Yield:	**Prep time:**	**Cook time:**	**Serving size:**
8 slices	15 minutes	35 minutes	1/8 loaf
Each serving has:			
144 calories	9 g carbohydrates	2 g fat	2 g fiber
17 g protein			

1 lb. 99 percent lean ground white turkey
1 cup mixed frozen vegetables
1/2 cup whole-wheat breadcrumbs
1/4 cup old-fashioned oats
1 tsp. dried oregano
2 large egg whites
1/2 cup fat-free shredded mozzarella cheese
1/2 tsp. salt
1/2 cup chopped fresh tarragon
2 TB. reduced-fat grated Parmesan cheese

1. Preheat the oven to 375°F. Line a 8 1/2×4 1/2×2 1/2-inch meatloaf pan with aluminum foil, and spray it with nonstick cooking spray.
2. In a large bowl, combine ground turkey, frozen vegetables, breadcrumbs, old-fashioned oats, oregano, egg whites, mozzarella cheese, salt, and tarragon. Transfer meat mixture to the prepared pan, and form into a loaf.
3. Sprinkle Parmesan cheese over meatloaf, and cover with another piece of aluminum foil. Bake for 25 minutes, remove the top aluminum foil, and bake for 10 more minutes.
4. Remove the pan from the oven, and cool for 5 minutes before serving.

TUMMY TAMER

Adding oats to lean ground meat retains moisture and adds some healthy fiber without altering the taste or flavor of the dish.

Colorful Turkey Burgers

Juicy, mouthwatering, and filling, these turkey burgers are a great substitute for fatty beef burgers—and are acid reflux friendly!

Yield:	**Prep time:**	**Cook time:**	**Serving size:**
4 burgers	20 minutes	15 minutes	1 burger
Each serving has:			
144 calories 11 g protein	18 g carbohydrates	4 g fat	3 g fiber

- 1 lb. 99 percent lean white ground turkey
- 1 cup quick-cooking oats
- 1 cup shredded carrot
- 1 cup diced zucchini
- ½ cup crumbled low-fat feta cheese
- ½ cup chopped fresh parsley
- 4 large egg whites

1. Spray a large skillet with nonstick cooking spray, and set over medium-high heat.
2. In a medium bowl, combine ground turkey, quick-cooking oats, carrot, zucchini, feta cheese, parsley, and egg whites.
3. Form mixture into 4 patties, and add to the preheated skillet. Cook for about 3 or 4 minutes per side or until an instant-read thermometer registers an internal temperature of 165°F.
4. Serve on whole-wheat buns or wrap in a fresh lettuce leaf.

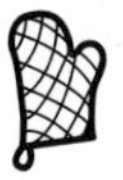

COOLER TALK

Since the 1970s, consumption of turkey has increased by 108 percent in the United States.

Cheesy Turkey Burger Delights

As you bite into these juicy turkey burgers, you'll find a cheesy surprise!

Yield:	**Prep time:**	**Cook time:**	**Serving size:**
4 burgers	10 minutes	15 minutes	1 burger
Each serving has:			
292 calories	14 g carbohydrates	10 g fat	2 g fiber
34 g protein			

1 lb. 99 percent lean ground turkey

1 large egg

1 cup whole-wheat breadcrumbs

1 tsp. fennel seeds

¼ tsp. salt

¼ cup chopped fresh parsley

3 oz. reduced-fat *Brie* cheese, roughly cubed

1. Spray a large skillet with nonstick cooking spray, and set over medium-high heat.
2. In a large bowl, combine ground turkey, egg, breadcrumbs, fennel seeds, salt, and parsley.
3. Form half of mixture into 4 thin patties. Top each patty with ¼ of Brie. Form another 4 thin patties, and top off burgers, sealing Brie inside.
4. Add all 4 burgers to the skillet, and cook for 2 minutes per side. Reduce heat to low, cover, and cook for 10 more minutes or until turkey is cooked through. Serve on a toasted whole-wheat bun or 2 green lettuce leaves.

DEFINITION

Brie is a creamy cow's milk cheese from France with a soft, edible rind and a mild flavor.

Apple-Sautéed Turkey Tenderloin

This dish nicely pairs the sweetness of apples and butternut squash with the flavor of the turkey. The meat retains lots of moisture and melts in your mouth.

Yield:	**Prep time:**	**Cook time:**	**Serving size:**
10 pieces	15 minutes	15 minutes	2 pieces
Each serving has:			
205 calories	7 g carbohydrates	5 g fat	1 g fiber
32 g protein			

1 TB. olive oil

1 TB. light butter

1 cup butternut squash, peeled and diced

1 apple (your favorite), cored and diced

$\frac{1}{4}$ tsp. salt

$\frac{1}{4}$ tsp. ground *coriander*

$1\frac{1}{2}$ lb. turkey tenderloin, cut into 1-in. medallions

1. In a medium skillet over medium-high heat, heat olive oil. Add light butter, butternut squash, apple, salt, and coriander, and cook for about 3 or 4 minutes or until lightly browned.
2. Add turkey, and cook for about 12 more minutes, turning every 3 or 4 minutes to brown all sides equally. If turkey is still rare inside, reduce heat to low, cover the skillet, and cook for a few more minutes or until turkey medallions are fully cooked and an instant-read thermometer reads 165°F.
3. Serve with baked potatoes, mashed potatoes, mashed cauliflower, or a side of steamed vegetables. If you want lower-calorie sides, stick to nonstarchy vegetables.

Variation: This dish can also be prepared with pork tenderloin instead of turkey tenderloin.

DEFINITION

Coriander is a rich, warm, spicy seed used in all types of recipes, from African to South American, from entrées to desserts.

Chicken Satay

This tender, palatable, tempting chicken is both sweet and savory.

Yield:	**Prep time:**	**Cook time:**	**Serving size:**
9 skewers	10 minutes, plus 30 minutes marinate time	25 minutes	3 skewers
Each serving has:			
361 calories	1 g carbohydrates	12 g fat	1 g fiber
59 g protein			

4 medium boneless, skinless chicken breasts, cut into 1-in. cubes

¼ tsp. salt

1 tsp. ground turmeric

1 tsp. ground coriander

1 tsp. ground cumin

1 tsp. ground cinnamon

1 TB. canola oil

1. In a medium bowl, combine chicken, salt, turmeric, coriander, cumin, cinnamon, and canola oil. Cover and refrigerate for at least 30 minutes.
2. Preheat the oven to 350°F.
3. Dip 9 skewers in water or lightly spray with cooking spray.
4. Remove chicken from marinade, and discard marinade. Place 3 cubes marinated chicken on each skewer, and place skewers on a baking sheet.
5. Bake for 25 minutes or until chicken is thoroughly cooked and an instant-read thermometer reads 165°F.

TUMMY TAMER

Wooden skewers need to be soaked in water, sprayed with nonstick cooking spray, or wrapped in aluminum foil on the exposed ends so they don't burn when exposed to high temperatures. You can also take all three of these precautionary measures.

Maple Ginger Chicken Joy

This sweet, zesty, and spicy dish is a wonderful protein-packed poultry treat.

Yield:	**Prep time:**	**Cook time:**	**Serving size:**
4 breasts	10 minutes, plus 4 hours or overnight marinate time	15 minutes	1 breast
Each serving has:			
365 calories 54 g protein	16 g carbohydrates	8 g fat	1 g fiber

2 TB. brown sugar

3 TB. maple syrup

$\frac{1}{4}$ tsp. fresh peeled and ground gingerroot

2 TB. sesame seeds

2 TB. low-sodium soy sauce

$\frac{1}{8}$ tsp. salt

4 (6- to 8-oz.) boneless, skinless chicken breasts

1. In a medium bowl, combine brown sugar, maple syrup, ground gingerroot, sesame seeds, soy sauce, and salt. Add chicken breasts, cover, and refrigerate for 4 hours or overnight.
2. Set a medium skillet over medium-high heat, and spray with nonstick cooking spray.
3. Remove chicken from marinade, and discard marinade. Add chicken breasts, and cook for 7 or 8 minutes on each side or until cooked through and an instant-read thermometer reads 165°F.

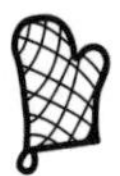

COOLER TALK

Other than color, there's no significant nutritional difference between white and brown sugar. Some studies show that brown sugar has more antioxidants. However, you'd need to eat lots of sugar to notice the difference in your diet. For optimal health, reduce the amount of added sugar you're consuming altogether.

Breaded Baked Chicken Tenders

Crispy on the outside and moist on the inside, these chicken tenders are a favorite of adults and kids alike.

Yield:	**Prep time:**	**Cook time:**	**Serving size:**
8 tenders	10 minutes	45 minutes	2 tenders
Each serving has:			
183 calories	15 g carbohydrates	9 g fat	1 g fiber
11 g protein			

2 large eggs, beaten

⅓ cup fresh parsley, chopped

1 cup panko breadcrumbs

4 TB. reduced-fat grated Parmesan cheese

8 chicken tenders

1. Preheat the oven to 350°F. Line a baking dish with aluminum foil, and spray it with nonstick cooking spray.
2. Pour eggs into a small bowl.
3. In a separate small bowl, combine parsley, breadcrumbs, and Parmesan cheese.
4. Dip chicken tenders, one at a time, into eggs and then into breadcrumb mixture to coat. Arrange in a single layer in the baking dish.
5. Bake for 45 minutes or until outside is golden brown and an instant-read thermometer reads 165°F. Flip one time midway through cooking.

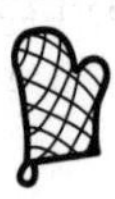

COOLER TALK

Egg color doesn't matter when it comes to the nutritional content. They're the same product, just in different packaging.

Chicken Kiev

This is a delicious twist on a dish traditionally stuffed with butter and herbs, yet it retains the flavor and moisture.

Yield:	**Prep time:**	**Cook time:**	**Serving size:**
4 breasts	15 minutes	35 minutes	1 breast
Each serving has:			
319 calories	13 g carbohydrates	10 g fat	1 g fiber
42 g protein			

$\frac{1}{2}$ cup fat-free cream cheese
2 TB. chopped fresh tarragon
2 TB. chopped fresh parsley
$\frac{1}{4}$ tsp. salt
2 large egg whites, beaten
4 (4-oz.) boneless, skinless chicken breasts
1 cup panko whole-wheat breadcrumbs

1. Preheat the oven to 375°F. Spray an 8×8-inch baking pan with nonstick cooking spray.
2. In a small dish, combine cream cheese, tarragon, parsley, and salt.
3. Pour egg whites into a small bowl.
4. Butterfly each chicken breast, cutting it in half lengthwise in the middle without cutting all the way through. Stuff each chicken breast with $\frac{1}{4}$ of cream cheese mixture.
5. Dip each stuffed chicken breast into egg whites and then into breadcrumbs to coat. Place in the baking pan, and bake for about 35 minutes or until an instant-read thermometer reads 165°F.

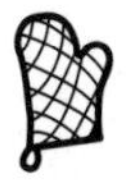

COOLER TALK

Authentic chicken Kiev is a dish high in fat with lots of butter and artery-clogging saturated fat. This version is much healthier, doesn't cause reflux—and, I dare say, tastes better, too!

Moroccan-Inspired Chicken

A captivating blend of cinnamon and ginger combined with a perfect contrast of pistachios and raisins will have your guests talking about this dish for a long time.

Yield:	**Prep time:**	**Cook time:**	**Serving size:**
4 cups	10 minutes	10 minutes	1 cup
Each serving has:			
187 calories	8 g carbohydrates	6 g fat	2 g fiber
26 g protein			

1 TB. olive oil

¼ tsp. ground ginger

¼ tsp. ground cinnamon

¼ tsp. salt

3 TB. shelled whole pistachios

1 cup shredded carrots

2 TB. raisins

1 lb. chicken breast cutlets, cut into 1-in. pieces

3 TB. water

1. In a medium skillet over medium-high heat, heat olive oil. Add ginger, cinnamon, salt, and pistachios, and mix well.
2. Add carrots and raisins, and cook for 1 or 2 minutes, stirring constantly to be sure they don't burn.
3. Quickly add chicken, and mix well so spices don't burn. Cook, stirring, for 5 more minutes.
4. Add water, cover, and set aside for 5 minutes before serving. Serve over rice or couscous.

TUMMY TAMER

Shredded carrots are available in your grocery store. Buying them shredded can save you time peeling and shredding.

Basil Chicken

The refreshing flavor of basil pairs beautifully with tender and juicy chicken in this recipe.

Yield:	**Prep time:**	**Cook time:**	**Serving size:**
6 breasts	10 minutes	35 minutes	1 breast
Each serving has:			
212 calories	7 g carbohydrates	3 g fat	1 g fiber
37 g protein			

3 cups fat-free milk

1 cup chopped fresh basil

½ tsp. salt

1½ cups fat-free shredded mozzarella cheese

6 (4-oz.) skinless chicken breasts

1. Preheat the oven to 375°F.
2. In a medium cast-iron skillet, combine fat-free milk, basil, salt, and mozzarella cheese.
3. Add chicken breasts, and bake for 35 minutes or until chicken is thoroughly cooked on the inside and no pink areas remain.

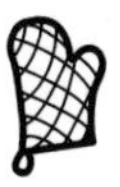

COOLER TALK

Milk has the property of tenderizing protein. Although the jury is still out, it has been found that the calcium in milk activates enzymes in meat that help break down proteins, producing a tender product.

Vegetarian Main Courses

Chapter

18

In This Chapter

- Mouthwatering homemade veggie burgers
- Protein-packed casseroles and stews
- Pizza, Parmesan, and other fun

How often do you stare at the frozen veggie burgers at the supermarket, wondering how complicated would it be to try making them yourself? I have great news for you—it's easy! Many veggie burgers are based around only a few ingredients that make them stick together—beans, flour, potatoes, and maybe a little bit of tahini paste. The rest is up to your imagination. In this chapter, you'll find some recipes to get you started. It's a great idea to make extras when you're cooking and freeze them for later.

Another dish you may not have thought of as being easy to make is pizza dough. It only requires mixing a couple ingredients together and is a fun activity for the entire family to do together. Because you're likely avoiding tomato sauce (a common acid reflux trigger), consider exploring some of the other toppings suggested in this chapter or creating your own flavor combinations.

Chickpea Veggie Burgers

Spiced just right and cooked to perfection, these juicy burger patties are packed with flavor and nutrients.

Yield:	**Prep time:**	**Cook time:**	**Serving size:**
8 burgers	15 minutes	20 minutes	1 burger
Each serving has:			
138 calories	21 g carbohydrates	4 g fat	5 g fiber
6 g protein			

1 TB. olive oil

1 cup shredded zucchini

1½ cups shredded carrots

¼ tsp. salt

1 tsp. ground cumin

1 (15-oz.) can *chickpeas,* drained and rinsed

¼ cup tahini paste

½ cup all-purpose flour

¼ cup chopped fresh parsley

1. In a medium skillet over medium-high heat, heat olive oil. Add zucchini, carrots, salt, and cumin, mix well, and cook for about 5 to 7 minutes or until vegetables are slightly soft and browned.
2. In a separate bowl, add chickpeas and tahini paste. Mash well or blend with a handheld blender. Add vegetables, flour, and parsley, and mix well. Form mixture into 8 patties.
3. In the same skillet over medium-high heat, cook patties for 7 or 8 minutes per side or until golden brown on the outside and cooked through on the inside.
4. Serve warm on a toasted bun, between 2 slices of bread, or with a baked potato.

DEFINITION

Chickpeas (also called garbanzo beans) are a yellow-gold, roundish bean that's the base ingredient in hummus. Chickpeas are high in fiber and low in fat, making them a delicious and healthful component of many appetizers and main dishes.

Portobello Mushroom Burgers

Light, yet savory, these meaty and juicy burgers will keep you full for a long time.

Yield:	**Prep time:**	**Cook time:**	**Serving size:**
2 burgers	10 minutes	10 minutes	1 burger
Each serving has:			
366 calories	36 g carbohydrates	19 g fat	6 g fiber
16 g protein			

1 TB. olive oil

2 large *portobello mushroom* caps

2 slices reduced-fat provolone cheese

$\frac{1}{2}$ cup roasted red peppers

$\frac{1}{2}$ medium avocado, peeled, seeded, and sliced thin

2 whole-wheat burger buns, toasted

1. In a medium skillet over medium-high heat, heat olive oil. Add portobello mushroom caps, and cook for 3 to 5 minutes per side until tender but not limp.
2. During the last minute of cooking, top each cap with 1 slice provolone cheese.
3. Place $\frac{1}{2}$ of roasted red peppers, 1 mushroom cap, and some avocado slices inside each burger bun, and serve warm.

DEFINITION

Portobello mushrooms are the mature and larger form of the smaller crimini mushroom. Portobellos are brownish, chewy, and flavorful. They're trendy served as whole caps, grilled, and as thin sautéed slices.

Vegetarian Edamame Stir-Fry

This flavorful stir-fry is great as a main dish or as a side. It also tastes great served over a small bowl of white rice.

Yield:	**Prep time:**	**Cook time:**	**Serving size:**
6 cups	10 minutes	20 minutes	$1\frac{1}{2}$ cups
Each serving has:			
212 calories	20 g carbohydrates	12 g fat	5 g fiber
10 g protein			

2 TB. sesame oil

1 cup shredded carrots

2 cups frozen edamame

1 cup frozen corn

1 cup bean sprouts

1 cup snow peas

$\frac{1}{4}$ tsp. salt

1 TB. low-sodium soy sauce

1 TB. white sesame seeds

1 TB. black sesame seeds

1. In a large saucepan over medium-high heat, heat sesame oil. Add carrots, and cook for 3 or 4 minutes. When carrots begin to soften, add edamame and corn. When edamame and corn have fully defrosted and are beginning to slightly brown (about 5 minutes), add bean sprouts and snow peas.
2. Season with salt, soy sauce, white sesame seeds, and black sesame seeds. Mix well, and serve warm.

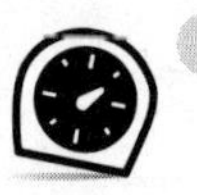

TUMMY TAMER

Edamame in pods makes a great snack. Full of fiber and protein, they'll keep you full for hours.

Quinoa Cakes

These cakes taste nutty and are a complete source of amino acids.

Yield:	**Prep time:**	**Cook time:**	**Serving size:**
6 cakes	15 minutes	10 minutes	2 cakes
Each serving has:			
331 calories	36 g carbohydrates	17 g fat	4 g fiber
12 g protein			

1 cup cooked whole-wheat quinoa
1 large egg
½ cup all-purpose flour
¼ cup tahini paste
2 TB. apple cider
¼ cup chopped fresh parsley
2 TB. chopped fresh dill
¼ tsp. salt
2 TB. shelled pumpkin seeds

1. In a medium bowl, combine whole-wheat quinoa, egg, flour, tahini paste, apple cider, parsley, dill, salt, and pumpkin seeds. Using a ⅓-cup measure, form mixture into 6 patties.
2. In a medium skillet over medium-high heat, cook patties for 5 minutes per side or until golden brown on the outside and cooked through on the inside.

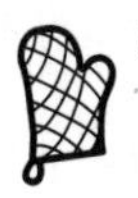

COOLER TALK

Quinoa is a great way to get protein in your diet if you're a vegetarian. It's a complete protein source and has all eight essential amino acids your body needs.

Vegetarian Bean Casserole

This flavorful and filling dish is perfect as an appetizer or a main course. The cheesiness and the flavors make this a perfect game-day treat.

Yield:	**Prep time:**	**Cook time:**	**Serving size:**
8 servings	15 minutes	25 minutes	1/8 recipe
Each serving has:			
303 calories	41 g carbohydrates	8 g fat	7 g fiber
18 g protein			

4 cups baked tortilla chips

1 (15-oz.) can black beans, drained and rinsed

1 medium avocado, peeled, seeded, and diced

1 cup canned corn

1/2 cup chopped fresh cilantro

1/4 cup chopped fresh parsley

1/2 tsp. salt

1 1/2 cups fat-free shredded mozzarella cheese

1 1/2 cups reduced-fat grated Parmesan cheese

1. Preheat the oven to 350°F. Spray an 8×8-inch baking dish with nonstick cooking spray.
2. Arrange tortilla chips in the prepared baking dish. Set aside.
3. In a medium bowl, combine black beans, avocado, corn, cilantro, parsley, and salt.
4. In a small bowl, combine mozzarella cheese and Parmesan cheese.
5. Sprinkle 1/3 of cheese mixture over tortillas, top with bean mixture, and continue layering, finishing with cheese mixture on top.
6. Bake, uncovered, for 25 minutes or until cheese is all melted and beans are heated through.

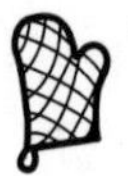

COOLER TALK

Beans are rich in fiber, protein, B vitamins, iron, phosphorous, magnesium, manganese, potassium, copper, calcium, and zinc. Incorporate them into your recipes and experiment with different types to add variety, flavor, and color to your meals.

Spinach and Mushroom Square Pizza

Perfectly baked crust with a delicious topping? Only one word is needed to describe the flavor—yum!

Yield:	**Prep time:**	**Cook time:**	**Serving size:**
6 slices	1 hour	15 minutes	1 slice
Each serving has:			
268 calories	43 g carbohydrates	6 g fat	4 g fiber
12 g protein			

2 TB. light butter
2 TB. plus 1 cup all-purpose flour
$\frac{1}{2}$ cup skim milk
$\frac{1}{2}$ cup low-fat chicken broth
1 (10-oz.) pkg. frozen spinach, thawed and squeezed
$1\frac{1}{2}$ cups chopped shiitake mushrooms
$\frac{3}{4}$ cup warm (110°F to 115°F) water
$\frac{1}{2}$ tsp. fast-acting dry yeast
$\frac{1}{2}$ tsp. honey
1 cup bread flour
2 TB. cornmeal
$\frac{1}{4}$ cup reduced-fat grated Parmesan cheese
$\frac{1}{2}$ cup fat-free shredded mozzarella cheese

1. In a medium skillet over medium-high heat, melt butter. Add 2 tablespoons all-purpose flour, and cook, stirring constantly, for 30 seconds to 1 minute. Slowly pour in skim milk and chicken broth, whisking to avoid clumps. Add spinach and shiitake mushrooms, mix well, and set aside.
2. In a small bowl, pour $\frac{1}{4}$ cup warm water. Add fast-acting dry yeast and honey, and mix well. Set aside for approximately 10 minutes to *proof.*
3. Meanwhile, lightly flour a countertop.
4. In a medium bowl, combine remaining 1 cup all-purpose flour, bread flour, and remaining $\frac{1}{2}$ cup warm water. Add yeast mixture. Turn out dough onto the floured counter, and knead for approximately 5 minutes.
5. Place dough back in the bowl, and cover with plastic wrap. Set the bowl in a warm place free of any drafts, and allow dough to rise for approximately 40 minutes.

6. Preheat the oven to 450°F. Sprinkle a cookie sheet with cornmeal.
7. Place dough on the cookie sheet, and roll out into a square. Set aside to rise for 15 more minutes.
8. Top pizza with mushroom mixture, Parmesan cheese, and mozzarella cheese. Bake for 12 to 15 minutes or until cheeses are melted and crust is golden brown.

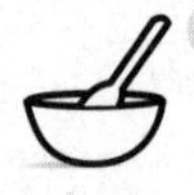

DEFINITION

To **proof** is to place yeast in warm water and allow it to start producing bubbly foam. This indicates the yeast is active.

Indian Pulao

This recipe has authentic Indian flavors and spices without any potential acid reflux triggers—yum!

Yield:	**Prep time:**	**Cook time:**	**Serving size:**
6 servings	15 minutes	50 minutes	1/6 recipe
Each serving has:			
292 calories	50 g carbohydrates	8 g fat	3 g fiber
6 g protein			

2 cups basmati rice

2 TB. olive oil

2 TB. cashews

1 TB. raisins

1 bay leaf

3 whole cardamoms

3 whole cloves

1/8 tsp. ground cinnamon

1 TB. freshly peeled and grated ginger

1 tsp. dried cilantro

1/4 tsp. salt

1 large carrot, peeled and diced

1/2 cup frozen green peas

1 cup cauliflower florets

1/2 tsp. ground turmeric

4 cups water

1. In a medium bowl, cover basmati rice with water, and soak for 30 minutes.
2. In a medium saucepan over medium-high heat, heat 1 tablespoon olive oil. Add cashews and raisins, and cook for about 3 or 4 minutes. Set aside.
3. In a medium skillet over medium-high heat, heat remaining 1 tablespoon olive oil. Add bay leaf, cardamoms, cloves, cinnamon, ginger, cilantro, and salt, and cook, stirring so spices don't burn.
4. Add carrot, peas, and cauliflower, and mix well. Cook for 5 to 10 minutes or until vegetables are tender. Add turmeric.
5. Add rice and 4 cups water, and stir well. Reduce heat to low, cover, and cook for about 30 to 40 minutes or until liquid is all absorbed and rice is fluffy.

6. When rice is ready, stir in cashews and raisins, and serve warm. Remove bay leaf before serving.

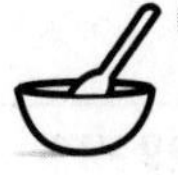

DEFINITION

Pulao is a rice dish that originated in the Far East. It's flavored with aromatic spices and varies depending on the region and country. Pilau and pilaf are sisters of pulao.

Corn and Pea Sabazi

The sweetness of the corn paired with the complex flavors of Indian spices creates rich and unforgettable flavor.

Yield:	**Prep time:**	**Cook time:**	**Serving size:**
2 wraps	5 minutes	10 minutes	1 wrap
Each serving has:			
441 calories	67 g carbohydrates	16 g fat	15 g fiber
16 g protein			

1 TB. olive oil

1 TB. dried cilantro

1 tsp. fresh peeled and grated ginger

2 whole cloves

1/2 tsp. ground turmeric

1/4 tsp. salt

1 cup frozen corn

1 cup frozen peas

1/2 cup canned chickpeas, drained and rinsed

2 medium whole-wheat wraps

1. In a medium skillet over medium-high heat, heat olive oil. Add cilantro flakes, ginger, cloves, turmeric, and salt, and cook for 30 seconds to 1 minute.
2. Add corn and peas, and stir well. Cook for about 7 or 8 minutes or until vegetables are defrosted and lightly browned.
3. Add chickpeas, and cook for 3 or 4 more minutes.
4. Divide vegetable mixture between 2 whole-wheat wraps, and serve.

Variation: Instead of wrapping, you can serve the vegetable mixture over rice.

DEFINITION

Sabazi is a word that collectively describes any vegetable dish in Indian cuisine.

Baked Sesame Tofu

This tofu dish is incredibly flavorful and goes well with rice, on sandwiches, or with potatoes.

Yield:	**Prep time:**	**Cook time:**	**Serving size:**
8 slices	10 minutes, plus 4 hours to overnight marinate time	20 minutes	2 slices
Each serving has:			
365 calories	6 g carbohydrates	34 g fat	2 g fiber
9 g protein			

1 tsp. fresh peeled and grated ginger

1 tsp. brown sugar

1/4 cup toasted sesame oil

1/4 cup peanut oil

3 TB. low-sodium soy sauce

1/8 tsp. salt

1/4 cup toasted sesame seeds

14 oz. firm tofu

1. In a medium bowl, combine ginger, brown sugar, toasted sesame oil, peanut oil, soy sauce, salt, and toasted sesame seeds.
2. Cut tofu into 8 equal slices. Add tofu to marinade, cover, and refrigerate for 4 hours to overnight.
3. Preheat the oven to 425°F. Coat a small baking dish with nonstick cooking spray.
4. Arrange tofu slices in a single layer in the baking dish, and bake for 17 to 20 minutes or until golden brown.

TUMMY TAMER

In addition to being a good source of protein, tofu has 200 to 330 milligrams calcium, depending on the brand.

Eggplant Parmesan

This delightful treat is so rich and creamy, no one will ever suspect how healthy it is.

Yield:	**Prep time:**	**Cook time:**	**Serving size:**
1 large eggplant	15 minutes	45 minutes	1/8 eggplant
Each serving has:			
176 calories	20 g carbohydrates	6 g fat	6 g fiber
12 g protein			

1 1/2 cups whole-wheat breadcrumbs

1/4 cup fresh curly parsley, chopped

1/4 cup fresh cilantro, chopped

1 cup fat-free ricotta cheese

1/8 tsp. dried basil

1/2 cup reduced-fat grated Parmesan cheese

1 cup fat-free shredded mozzarella cheese

1 large egg

3 large egg whites

2 large eggplants, thinly sliced lengthwise

1. Preheat the oven to 375°F. Spray a 9×13-inch baking pan with nonstick cooking spray.
2. In a medium bowl, combine breadcrumbs, parsley, and cilantro. Set aside.
3. In a small bowl, combine ricotta cheese and basil. Set aside.
4. In another small bowl, combine Parmesan cheese and mozzarella cheese. Set aside.
5. In a medium bowl, whisk egg and egg whites.
6. Dip eggplant slices, one at a time, into egg mixture, and layer on the bottom of the baking dish. Top with ricotta mixture, and add another layer of breaded eggplant. Sprinkle some of cheese mixture on top, and repeat layering, finishing off with cheese on top.

7. Bake for approximately 45 minutes or until eggplant slices are baked through and golden brown on top.

TUMMY TAMER

If you have extra time, consider sweating the eggplant by sautéing it for several minutes, covering the pan with a lid, and sweating for about 5 minutes. This will extract more flavors that will take your dish to the next level.

Perfect Pastas and Grains

Chapter 19

In This Chapter

- Versatile pasta dishes
- Creamy, cheesy comfort foods
- Rice, couscous, and other grains

If you like pasta, start boiling your water! This chapter doesn't disappoint, with mouthwatering creamy linguini and oven-baked macaroni and cheese. The following pages feature a variety of grain recipes rich in color and nutrients. Whole grains are high in B vitamins, vitamin E, magnesium, zinc, and copper and are also a good source of fiber.

Consider having fun with your grains and experimenting with those you've never tried before.

Bowtie and Buckwheat Pasta

This traditional dish combines two grains that both have sweet and comforting undertones.

Yield:	**Prep time:**	**Cook time:**	**Serving size:**
6 cups	10 minutes	22 minutes	1/3 cup
Each serving has:			
101 calories	13 g carbohydrates	4 g fat	1 g fiber
3 g protein			

3 cups water
1/2 tsp. salt
1 cup bowtie pasta
1/2 cup buckwheat
2 TB. olive oil
3 TB. grated Parmesan cheese

1. In a medium saucepan over high heat, bring 2 cups water to a boil. Add 1/4 teaspoon salt and bowtie pasta, and cook for about 6 to 8 minutes or until pasta is al dente. Drain pasta in a colander.
2. In a separate medium saucepan over high heat, bring remaining 1 cup water to a boil. Add buckwheat and remaining 1/4 teaspoon salt. Return to a boil, reduce heat to medium-low, cover, and simmer for about 10 minutes or until water is absorbed.
3. In a medium skillet over high heat, heat olive oil. Add bowtie pasta, and cook for about 4 minutes or until lightly browned. Add buckwheat, and mix thoroughly. Sprinkle with Parmesan cheese, and serve.

TUMMY TAMER

Buckwheat is not only gluten free, but it also contains all eight essential amino acids, making it a great source of protein. You find buckwheat in the supermarket among other grains such as rice, millet, and quinoa.

Baked Macaroni and Cheese

This classic comfort food contains so much cheesy goodness, you'll have a hard time saying no to seconds.

Yield:	**Prep time:**	**Cook time:**	**Serving size:**
$10\frac{1}{2}$ cups	10 minutes	30 minutes	$1\frac{3}{4}$ cups
Each serving has:			
383 calories	64 g carbohydrates	6 g fat	3 g fiber
16 g protein			

1 (16-oz.) pkg. penne rigate pasta

2 TB. light butter

2 TB. all-purpose flour

1 cup skim milk

1 tsp. salt

$\frac{1}{2}$ cup reduced-fat grated Parmesan cheese

$\frac{1}{2}$ cup fat-free shredded mozzarella cheese

$\frac{1}{2}$ cup whole-wheat breadcrumbs

1. Preheat the oven to 400°F. Spray a baking pan with nonstick spray.
2. Cook pasta according to the package directions until *al dente*. Remove from heat, drain, and return pasta to the cooking pot.
3. In a large skillet over medium-high heat, melt light butter. Whisk in all-purpose flour, and cook for 1 minute or until lightly brown.
4. Gradually pour in skim milk, whisking to avoid clumps. Add salt, Parmesan cheese, and mozzarella cheese.
5. Pour cheese mixture over prepared pasta, and spread pasta mixture in the prepared baking pan. Evenly top with breadcrumbs.
6. Bake for about 20 minutes or until top is golden brown.

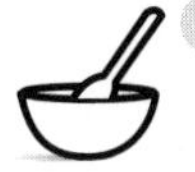

DEFINITION

Al dente is Italian for "against the teeth." The term refers to pasta (or another ingredient such as rice) that's neither soft nor hard but just slightly firm against the teeth. This, according to many pasta aficionados, is the perfect way to cook pasta.

Creamy Linguini with Peas

This cheesy and creamy dish features sweet peas that pop in your mouth.

Yield:	**Prep time:**	**Cook time:**	**Serving size:**
7 cups	5 minutes	15 minutes	$1\frac{3}{4}$ cups
Each serving has:			
325 calories	42 g carbohydrates	10 g fat	7 g fiber
17 g protein			

$\frac{1}{2}$ lb. linguine

2 TB. light butter

$1\frac{1}{2}$ cups frozen baby peas

2 TB. all-purpose flour

$1\frac{1}{2}$ cups fat-free milk

$\frac{1}{2}$ cup reduced-fat grated Parmesan cheese

$\frac{1}{2}$ tsp. salt

$\frac{1}{2}$ cup chopped fresh parsley

1. Cook linguine according to the package directions until al dente. Drain, and rinse with cold water. Set aside.
2. In a medium skillet over high heat, melt butter. Add baby peas, and cook for 5 to 7 minutes or until peas are thawed and slightly browned on the outside.
3. Reduce heat to medium-high, add all-purpose flour, mix well, and cook for 30 seconds to 1 minute.
4. Slowly whisk in fat-free milk followed by Parmesan cheese. Add salt. Add pasta and parsley, mix well, and serve.

TUMMY TAMER

Parsley is a rich source of vitamin K and is only about 2 calories per tablespoon.

Saffron Risotto

Saffron adds a decadent flavor to this already rich dish.

Yield:	**Prep time:**	**Cook time:**	**Serving size:**
4 cups	10 minutes	30 minutes	1 cup
Each serving has:			
187 calories	32 g carbohydrates	3 g fat	2 g fiber
5 g protein			

3 cups vegetable stock

4 cups small broccoli florets

¼ tsp. saffron

1 TB. olive oil

¾ cup arborio rice

1. In a medium saucepan over high heat, bring vegetable stock to a simmer. Add broccoli florets, and cook for 2 or 3 minutes. Using a slotted spoon, remove broccoli and set aside.
2. Stir ⅛ teaspoon saffron into vegetable stock, reduce heat to low, and cover.
3. Meanwhile, in another medium saucepan over medium heat, heat olive oil. Add arborio rice, and sauté for 3 to 5 minutes.
4. Stir in 1 cup vegetable stock from the pan, reduce heat to medium-low, and cook, stirring regularly, until most of liquid is absorbed. Continue adding stock, ½ cup at a time, and stirring, for about 10 minutes or until liquid is absorbed.
5. Stir in remaining ⅛ teaspoon saffron before last addition of stock, and cook until most of liquid is absorbed.
6. Remove from heat, and stir in broccoli. Cover and let stand for 2 or 3 minutes before serving.

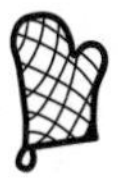

COOLER TALK

Saffron is the most expensive spice in the world. But it's so flavorful, you need only a small amount to flavor a large dish.

Cheesy Mushroom Quinoa

The nutty flavor of quinoa pairs nicely with the cheese and mushrooms in this dish.

Yield:	**Prep time:**	**Cook time:**	**Serving size:**
12 cups	10 minutes	25 minutes	½ cup
Each serving has:			
142 calories	20 g carbohydrates	5 g fat	3 g fiber
5 g protein			

1 cup quinoa, rinsed and drained

2 cups water

1 TB. extra-virgin olive oil

2 large portobello mushroom caps, diced

⅛ tsp. salt

¼ cup reduced-fat grated Parmesan cheese

¼ cup chopped fresh parsley

1. In a medium saucepan over high heat, bring quinoa and water to a boil. Reduce heat to low, cover, and cook for about 15 minutes or until water is absorbed.
2. Meanwhile, in a medium skillet over medium-high heat, heat extra-virgin olive oil. Add portobello mushrooms and salt, and cook, stirring frequently, for about 5 minutes.
3. Add cooked quinoa, Parmesan cheese, and parsley to the skillet, mix well, and serve warm.

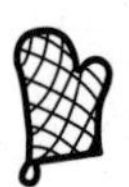

COOLER TALK

One portobello mushroom has more potassium than a glass of orange juice or a banana.

Couscous with Carrots and Almonds

This fun and colorful dish packs lots of flavor, thanks to the carrots along with the nice crunch of almonds.

Yield:	**Prep time:**	**Cook time:**	**Serving size:**
4 cups	5 minutes	10 minutes	1 cup
Each serving has:			
242 calories	40 g carbohydrates	5 g fat	4 g fiber
8 g protein			

1¾ cups vegetable stock

1 cup *couscous*

¾ cup shredded carrots

¼ cup toasted slivered almonds

¼ tsp. salt

1 TB. light butter

4 tsp. chopped fresh parsley (optional)

1. In a medium saucepan over high heat, bring vegetable stock to a boil. Remove from heat, and add couscous, carrots, almonds, and salt. Add light butter, and mix well.
2. Cover and allow to stand for 5 or 6 minutes or until liquid is all absorbed.
3. Separate into 4 bowls, garnish with parsley (if using), and serve.

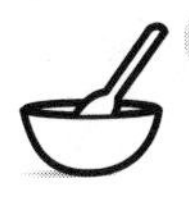

DEFINITION

Couscous is granular semolina (durum wheat) used in many Mediterranean and North African dishes. You can find couscous in the supermarket among all other grains. It's great as a quick side for weeknight meals or as a base for cold salads.

Colorful Couscous

This dish is tender on the palate and very rich in flavor. It has color, taste, and lots of healthy ingredients such as protein and fiber.

Yield:	**Prep time:**	**Cook time:**	**Serving size:**
$1\frac{1}{3}$ cups	15 minutes	15 minutes	$\frac{1}{3}$ cup
Each serving has:			
390 calories	75 g carbohydrates	5 g fat	14 g fiber
15 g protein			

1 TB. olive oil

$\frac{3}{4}$ cup shredded zucchini

$1\frac{1}{2}$ cups shredded carrots

$\frac{1}{4}$ tsp. salt

$\frac{1}{4}$ tsp. ground cumin

1 (15-oz.) can chickpeas, drained and rinsed

2 cups water

$1\frac{1}{4}$ cups whole-wheat couscous

1. In a large pot over medium-high heat, heat olive oil. Add zucchini, carrots, salt, and cumin, and cook, stirring constantly, for 3 minutes.
2. Add chickpeas, and cook, stirring occasionally, for about 2 more minutes.
3. In a small saucepan over high heat, bring water to boil.
4. Add couscous and boiling water to the large pot with vegetables. Mix well, remove from heat, cover, and set aside for about 5 minutes or until all water is absorbed and couscous is completely cooked. Serve warm.

TUMMY TAMER

To diversify your dish, use different varieties of couscous, including Moroccan (grains are the size of coarse salt) or Israeli (grains are the size of peppercorns).

Rice with Dates and Parsley

This dish has it all—it's chewy, sweet, and has just the right twist of savory.

Yield:	**Prep time:**	**Cook time:**	**Serving size:**
4 cups	10 minutes	30 minutes	1 cup
Each serving has:			
418 calories	85 g carbohydrates	5 g fat	3 g fiber
8 g protein			

4 cups water

2 cups white rice

$\frac{1}{4}$ tsp. salt

$\frac{1}{3}$ cup chopped dates

1 TB. light butter

2 TB. pine nuts

$\frac{1}{4}$ cup chopped fresh parsley

1. In a medium pot over high heat, bring water to a boil. Add white rice and salt, and cook for about 20 to 25 minutes or until all liquid is absorbed and rice is soft.
2. Add dates, light butter, pine nuts, and parsley. Mix well, and serve warm.

TUMMY TAMER

Dates are a rich source of potassium, iron, vitamin B_{12}, and niacin, making them a great snack alternative.

Rainbow Coconut Rice

With coconut undertones combined with the sweetness of colorful vegetables, this dish is both delicious to the palate and pleasing to the eye.

Yield:	**Prep time:**	**Cook time:**	**Serving size:**
10 cups	10 minutes	25 minutes	1⅔ cups
Each serving has:			
298 calories 5 g protein	53 g carbohydrates	7 g fat	3 g fiber

2 cups 50 percent reduced-fat coconut milk

2 cups water

¼ tsp. salt

2 cups basmati rice

¼ cup finely diced carrots

1 cup diced butternut squash

½ cup canned or frozen baby green peas

½ cup canned corn

2 TB. unsweetened shredded coconut flakes

1. In a medium pot over medium-high heat, bring coconut milk and water to a boil. Add salt and basmati rice, and bring back to a boil.
2. Add carrots and butternut squash, reduce heat to low, cover, and simmer for about 20 minutes or until almost all water is absorbed and rice is fluffy.
3. Add peas, corn, and coconut flakes. Cover and let stand for 5 more minutes or until remaining water is absorbed. Serve warm.

TUMMY TAMER

Make extra of this recipe, and freeze individual portions for quick and convenient meals later in the week.

Rice Pilaf

This *pilaf* is rich, flavorful, and creamy. The rice absorbs the flavor and aroma of the chicken, and the carrots add color.

Yield:	**Prep time:**	**Cook time:**	**Serving size:**
8 cups	5 minutes	1 hour	1 cup
Each serving has:			
255 calories	37 g carbohydrates	6 g fat	2 g fiber
12 g protein			

- 1 TB. olive oil
- 5 chicken drumsticks, with skin
- 2½ cups julienned carrots
- 4 cups water
- 2 cups basmati rice
- 1 tsp. salt
- 5 large bay leaves
- 1 tsp. ground cumin
- ¼ tsp. ground turmeric

1. In a large saucepan over medium heat, heat olive oil. Add drumsticks, and cook for 3 to 5 minutes or until lightly browned on all sides. Add carrots, and cook for 1 or 2 more minutes.
2. Add water, and bring to a boil. Add basmati rice and salt, and bring back to a boil.
3. Add bay leaves, cumin, and turmeric. Reduce heat to low, cover, and cook for 30 to 45 minutes. Remove bay leaves before serving.

Variation: Serve rice with or without the chicken. The main reason for using drumsticks in this dish is the incredible flavor and aroma they bring to the rice.

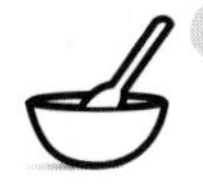

DEFINITION

Pilaf is a rice dish in which the rice is browned in butter or oil and then cooked in a flavorful liquid such as a broth, often with the addition of meats or vegetables. The rice absorbs the broth, resulting in a very savory dish.

Chapter 20

Vegetables on the Side

In This Chapter

- Superb spuds
- Veggie fries and mashes
- Colorful veggie fare for all palates

Veggies are an excellent way to add nutritious variety to your diet. Say good-bye to the old soggy veggies that may have turned you off to these nutritional powerhouses. The veg dishes in this chapter will keep boredom far away and introduce you to new colors and textures that will keep you coming back for seconds.

Oven-baked french fries, creamed spinach, and truffled mashed potatoes are healthy remakes of favorite comfort foods. They can make a great accompaniment to a weeknight dinner or become part of your holiday celebration.

The assortment of roasted veggie recipes in this chapter can make perfect side dishes, succulent appetizers, or ideal in-between-meal snacks. Leave them out on the table so you'll be more likely to grab a bite when you're passing by. Are you ready to turn on the oven and start cooking?

Truffled Mashed Potatoes

Truffle oil makes simple and routine mashed potatoes feel decadent and exquisite.

Yield:	Prep time:	Cook time:	Serving size:
3 cups	5 minutes	30 minutes	³⁄₄ cup
Each serving has:			
201 calories	33 g carbohydrates	3 g fat	4 g fiber
11 g protein			

6 to 8 Yukon Gold potatoes

1 TB. light butter

³⁄₄ cup fat-free cream

¹⁄₂ tsp. salt

1 tsp. white truffle oil

1. Place potatoes in a medium saucepan, cover with water, and set over high heat. Bring to a boil, reduce heat to medium, and cook for about 20 to 25 minutes or until potatoes are fork-tender.
2. Remove from heat, and pour out water. Add light butter, fat-free cream, salt, and white truffle oil, and mash well. Divide in 4 equal portions, and serve.

Variation: For variety, substitute black truffle oil for the white kind.

TUMMY TAMER

Truffle oil is more expensive than many other oil varieties. To compensate, it is so rich in flavor, you only need a tiny amount to add an incredible flavor to the dish. Consider investing in a small bottle and using it in both hot and cold dishes.

Oven-Baked Fries

These fries are crispy on the outside and soft on the inside—just like perfect fries should be.

Yield: 3 cups	**Prep time:** 10 minutes	**Cook time:** 45 minutes	**Serving size:** ½ cup
Each serving has: 202 calories 4 g protein	32 g carbohydrates	7 g fat	4 g fiber

6 large baking potatoes

3 TB. olive oil

½ tsp. salt

2 TB. dried rosemary

1. Preheat the oven to 425°F. Spray a baking pan with nonstick cooking spray.
2. Cut potatoes into french fries, and place on the prepared baking pan. Add olive oil, salt, and rosemary, and mix well to coat.
3. Bake for 45 minutes or until potatoes are golden brown and baked through.

TUMMY TAMER

Rosemary is an excellent source of folic acid, pyridoxine, vitamin A, and iron. If all possible, choose fresh rosemary over dried. Store fresh rosemary in the refrigerator in a sealed plastic bag for maximum shelf life.

Turnip Fries

If you like french fries, these surprisingly yummy, crispy, and cheesy bites might be just the right treat for you.

Yield: 16 cups	**Prep time:** 5 minutes	**Cook time:** 25 minutes	**Serving size:** 4 cups
Each serving has: 226 calories	29 g carbohydrates	11 g fat	8 g fiber
5 g protein			

12 medium turnips

3 TB. extra-virgin olive oil

¼ tsp. salt

3 TB. reduced-fat grated Parmesan cheese

1. Preheat the oven to 425°F.
2. Using a vegetable peeler, peel turnips. Cut them into french fries, and place on a 9×13-inch baking sheet. Add extra-virgin olive oil, salt, and Parmesan cheese, and toss well to coat.
3. Bake for 20 to 25 minutes, tossing once during baking to ensure even browning, or until fries turn golden brown.

TUMMY TAMER

Turnips are a great low-calorie, high-volume food. One cup cubed contains only 36 calories! As an added bonus, turnips are also high in vitamin C and fiber.

Rutabaga Purée

This silky dish tastes very similar to mashed potatoes and is a great way to load up on vegetables.

Yield:	**Prep time:**	**Cook time:**	**Serving size:**
8 cups	5 minutes	40 minutes	2 cups
Each serving has:			
139 calories 4 g protein	23 g carbohydrates	5 g fat	7 g fiber

10 to 12 medium *rutabaga,* peeled and roughly chopped

¼ tsp. salt

3 TB. light butter

¼ cup chopped fresh parsley

1. Place rutabaga in a medium saucepan, cover with water, and set over high heat. Bring to a boil, reduce heat to medium-low, and cook for about 30 minutes or until rutabaga is fork-tender.
2. Pour out water. Add salt, light butter, and parsley. Mash well, and serve.

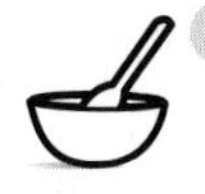

DEFINITION

Rutabagas, often confused for turnips, are a close relative of turnips, but technically they're a mix of turnips and cabbage.

Zucchini Pancakes

These crunchy on the outside and moist on the inside pancakes combine the freshness of summer with the warmth and the texture of the flour-based pancakes you know and love.

Yield:	**Prep time:**	**Cook time:**	**Serving size:**
8 pancakes	10 minutes	6 minutes	2 pancakes
Each serving has:			
189 calories	30 g carbohydrates	3 g fat	3 g fiber
9 g protein			

4 medium zucchini

2 medium eggs

1 cup *all-purpose flour*

2 TB. reduced-fat grated Parmesan cheese

1 TB. chopped fresh parsley

$\frac{1}{2}$ tsp. salt

2 TB. olive oil

1. Using a grater, shred zucchini into a large bowl. Squeeze to extract excess liquid if any accumulates in the bowl during the grating process, and discard liquid.
2. Add eggs, all-purpose flour, Parmesan cheese, parsley, and salt, and mix well. Form mixture into 8 pancakes.
3. In a large skillet over medium-high heat, heat olive oil. Add pancakes, and cook for 2 or 3 minutes per side or until golden brown and cooked through on the inside.

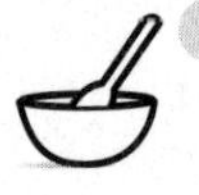

DEFINITION

All-purpose flour is flour that contains only the inner part of the wheat grain. It's suitable for all purposes, from cakes to gravies.

Cumin-Roasted Cauliflower

The crunchy texture and nutty and peppery flavor of this surprisingly delicious cauliflower will leave you satisfied for hours.

Yield:	**Prep time:**	**Cook time:**	**Serving size:**
6 cups	10 minutes	25 minutes	1 cup
Each serving has:			
54 calories	3 g carbohydrates	5 g fat	1 g fiber
1 g protein			

1 large head cauliflower, chopped into 1-in. florets

2 TB. olive oil

½ tsp. salt

1 tsp. cumin

1. Preheat the oven to 450°F.
2. In a large bowl, combine cauliflower florets, olive oil, salt, and cumin.
3. Transfer cauliflower to a cookie sheet, and spread into a single layer.
4. Roast for 25 minutes. Remove the tray from the oven, and set aside for 1 or 2 minutes before serving.

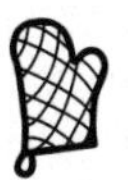

COOLER TALK

Almost all cauliflower in the United States comes from California. For only 25 calories per cup, this cruciferous vegetable is a great source of vitamin C, vitamin A, and folic acid.

Creamed Spinach

This healthy version of the old-time favorite tastes just like the real deal without the extra added fat and calories.

Yield:	**Prep time:**	**Cook time:**	**Serving size:**
2 cups	10 minutes	10 minutes	¼ cup
Each serving has:			
50 calories	5 g carbohydrates	3 g fat	1 g fiber
3 g protein			

2 TB. light butter

2 TB. all-purpose flour

1 cup low-sodium chicken broth

½ cup skim milk

1 (10-oz.) pkg. frozen spinach, thawed and drained

⅛ tsp. salt

1 TB. pine nuts

1. In a medium skillet over medium-high heat, melt light butter. Add flour, and cook for 1 or 2 minutes.
2. Slowly add chicken broth, whisking to avoid clumps. Slowly add skim milk, whisking to avoid clumps.
3. Add spinach, salt, and pine nuts, and mix well. Remove from heat, and serve warm.

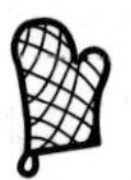

COOLER TALK

Three main types of spinach are sold in the United States: savoy, flat, and semi-savoy. Savoy stands for curly.

Simple Asian Stir-Fry

This *stir-fry* has a delicious sesame flavor and takes only minutes to prepare.

Yield:	**Prep time:**	**Cook time:**	**Serving size:**
5 cups	5 minutes	10 minutes	$1\frac{1}{3}$ cups
Each serving has:			
181 calories	18 g carbohydrates	10 g fat	6 g fiber
5 g protein			

2 TB. peanut oil

2 TB. low-sodium soy sauce

1 (1-lb.) bag frozen mixed vegetables

1 tsp. ground ginger

$\frac{1}{4}$ tsp. salt

1 tsp. toasted sesame oil

$2\frac{1}{2}$ TB. sesame seeds

1 tsp. cornstarch dissolved in 1 TB. water

1. In a large skillet over medium-high heat, heat peanut oil. Add soy sauce and frozen mixed vegetables, and cook for 5 to 7 minutes or until vegetables are fully thawed and golden brown on the outside.
2. Add ginger, salt, toasted sesame oil, and sesame seeds, and mix well.
3. Add cornstarch dissolved in water, and mix well to coat all ingredients. Cook for 1 or 2 more minutes. Remove from heat, and serve.

DEFINITION

To **stir-fry** is to cook small pieces of food in a wok or skillet over high heat, moving and turning the food quickly to cook all sides. A dished cooked by this method is also called a stir-fry.

Ginger Carrots

The ginger in this recipe nicely complements the sweetness of the carrots.

Yield: 4 cups	**Prep time:** 2 minutes	**Cook time:** 10 minutes	**Serving size:** 1 cup
Each serving has: 79 calories	13 g carbohydrates	3 g fat	4 g fiber
1 g protein			

4 cups baby carrots

2 TB. light butter

1 TB. brown sugar

¼ tsp. ground ginger

1. Place carrots in a medium saucepan, cover with water, and set over high heat. Bring to a boil, reduce heat to medium, and cook for about 25 minutes or until carrots are fork-tender.
2. In a medium saucepan over medium heat, melt light butter. Stir in brown sugar and ginger, and cook, stirring constantly, for 3 to 5 minutes or until sugar is dissolved.
3. Add carrots, stir gently until carrots are heated, and serve warm.

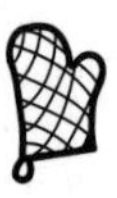

COOLER TALK

In ninth-century Europe, ground ginger had its place on the table alongside salt and pepper.

Sweet Potato Casserole

This sweet and rich comfort food makes a great addition to the Thanksgiving table.

Yield: 6 servings	**Prep time:** 15 minutes	**Cook time:** 1 hour	**Serving size:** 1/6 casserole
Each serving has: 334 calories 6 g protein	37 g carbohydrates	19 g fat	4 g fiber

2 large sweet potatoes, cubed
1/2 cup sugar
2 large eggs, beaten
1/2 tsp. salt
4 TB. light butter, softened
1/2 cup fat-free milk
1/2 tsp. vanilla extract
1/2 cup brown sugar
1/3 cup all-purpose flour
3 TB. light butter
1/2 cup chopped pecans

1. Preheat the oven to 325°F.
2. Place sweet potatoes in a medium saucepan, cover with water, and set over high heat. Bring to a boil, reduce heat to medium, cover, and cook for about 30 minutes or until sweet potatoes are fork-tender. Drain and mash lightly.
3. In a large bowl, combine sweet potatoes, sugar, eggs, salt, 4 tablespoons butter, fat-free milk, and vanilla extract. Transfer to a 9×13-inch baking dish.
4. In a medium bowl, combine brown sugar and all-purpose flour. Cut in light butter until mixture is slightly lumpy. Stir in pecans. Sprinkle mixture on top of sweet potato mixture in the baking dish.
5. Bake for 30 minutes or until golden brown in color.

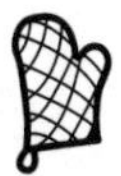

COOLER TALK

The sweet potato is a nutritional powerhouse, containing plenty of vitamin A, vitamin C, iron, and calcium. Sweet potatoes also contain an enzyme that converts starches into sugars, making them sweeter over time.

Roasted Acorn Squash

The sweetness of the brown sugar nicely complements the flavor of the acorn squash.

Yield:	**Prep time:**	**Cook time:**	**Serving size:**
2 acorn squash halves	10 minutes	1 to $1\frac{1}{2}$ hours	$\frac{1}{2}$ acorn squash
Each serving has:			
164 calories	36 g carbohydrates	3 g fat	3 g fiber
2 g protein			

1 medium acorn squash
1 TB. light butter
2 TB. maple syrup
$\frac{1}{4}$ tsp. ground cinnamon
$\frac{1}{4}$ cup water

1. Preheat the oven to 400°F.
2. Cut acorn squash in two, and scoop out seeds.
3. Spread light butter and maple syrup equally between halves. Sprinkle with cinnamon.
4. Place squash in a baking pan, and pour water into the bottom of the pan to avoid sticking and burning. Bake for 1 to $1\frac{1}{2}$ hours or until squash is soft and golden brown. Cool before serving.

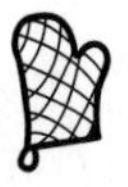

COOLER TALK

Squash come in many sizes, ranging from 10 to a whopping 600 pounds per squash.

Roasted Brussels Sprouts and Beets

Brussels sprouts and beets nicely complement each other for a decadent and flavorful dish.

Yield:	Prep time:	Cook time:	Serving size:
4 cups	10 minutes	40 minutes	$\frac{1}{2}$ cup
Each serving has:			
87 calories	6 g carbohydrates	7 g fat	2 g fiber
1 g protein			

2 cups brussels sprouts, cut in half

2 large red beets, cut into $\frac{1}{4}$-in. wedges

2 medium golden beets, cut into $\frac{1}{4}$-in. wedges

2 tsp. sea salt

4 TB. extra-virgin olive oil

1. Preheat the oven to 350°F.
2. In a large bowl, combine brussels sprouts, red beets, golden beets, sea salt, and extra-virgin olive oil.
3. Transfer vegetable mixture to a nonstick baking sheet, and roast for 40 minutes.

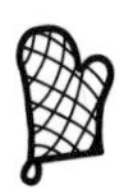

COOLER TALK

Brussels sprouts are rich in flavor and contain only 60 calories per cup. An added benefit: they're also an excellent source of vitamins K and C.

Chapter 21

Delectable Desserts

In This Chapter

- Melt-in-your-mouth cakes and pies
- Fruit desserts for all occasions
- Tasty cookies

A little sweet treat is a perfect way to finish a meal, to share love during the holidays (or any day!), and to satisfy a sweet tooth. This chapter is filled with mouthwatering recipes for all tastes and seasons.

Cakes, pies, and cookies are ideal for any celebration or weeknight meal and even can be frozen for later use. The fresh fruit salad and the fruit kebobs make a perfect dessert for a summer picnic or barbecue.

So let's get baking! Be sure to share the fruits of your labor with your entire family because the recipes in this chapter are healthy and loaded with good-for-you nutrients!

Creamy Cheesecake

Creamy, sweet, and smooth—just what you would expect from a perfect cheesecake.

Yield:	**Prep time:**	**Cook time:**	**Serving size:**
1 (9-inch) cheesecake	10 minutes	1 hour	⅛ cheesecake
Each serving has:			
245 calories	42 g carbohydrates	1 g fat	0 g fiber
17 g protein			

¼ cup graham cracker crumbs

3 (8-oz.) pkg. fat-free cream cheese

2 large eggs

1 cup fat-free Greek yogurt

1 cup sugar

1 tsp. vanilla extract

½ cup cake flour, sifted

1. Preheat the oven to 325°F.
2. Line the bottom of a 9-inch round baking pan with graham cracker crumbs. You can pat down the crumbs so they stick and form a crust if you like.
3. In a large bowl, combine cream cheese, eggs, Greek yogurt, sugar, and vanilla extract. With an electric mixer on medium, blend for 2 minutes or until smooth. Add cake flour, and blend for 1 more minute. Transfer cream cheese mixture to the baking pan.
4. Bake for 1 hour. Remove from the oven, and cool completely before serving.

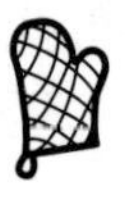

COOLER TALK

Believe it or not, vanilla extract has an indefinite shelf life, and its flavor is enhanced with time. Store in a cool, dark, and dry place.

Pumpkin Tart

If you love pumpkin, this tart is for you. It's slightly sweet, perfectly creamy, and has a hint of cinnamon.

Yield:	**Prep time:**	**Cook time:**	**Serving size:**
1 (9-inch) tart	10 minutes	35 minutes	⅛ tart
Each serving has:			
156 calories	31 g carbohydrates	1 g fat	2 g fiber
7 g protein			

¼ cup graham cracker crumbs

1 cup fat-free cream cheese

¾ cup sugar

1 (15-oz.) can unsweetened pumpkin purée

4 large egg whites

2 TB. maple syrup

1 tsp. vanilla extract

¼ tsp. salt

¼ tsp. ground cinnamon

1. Preheat the oven to 350°F.
2. Line the bottom of a 9-inch round baking pan with graham cracker crumbs.
3. In a large bowl, combine cream cheese, sugar, pumpkin purée, egg whites, maple syrup, vanilla extract, salt, and ground cinnamon. With an electric mixer on medium, blend for 3 minutes or until smooth. Transfer cream cheese mixture to the baking pan.
4. Bake for 35 minutes. Remove from the oven, and cool completely before serving. Serve in wedges with a dollop of reduced-fat whipped cream, vanilla frozen yogurt, or fat-free vanilla yogurt.

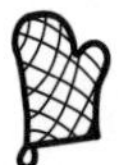

COOLER TALK

Pumpkin is a fat-free food that's low in calories and high in vitamin A. It's also your friend if you're looking for vitamin C and potassium. Unsweetened pumpkin purée can be used in cakes, pies, soups, and other dishes.

Angel Food Cake with Berries

The lightness of this angel food cake combines nicely with the sweetness of blackberries and blueberries.

Yield:	**Prep time:**	**Cook time:**	**Serving size:**
1 cake plus 5 cups berries	10 minutes	10 minutes	½ cup berries plus 1-inch slice angel food cake
Each serving has:			
157 calories	37 g carbohydrates	1 g fat	4 g fiber
3 g protein			

4 TB. sugar

2 TB. cornstarch

¼ tsp. ground cinnamon

2 TB. apple juice

1 cup water

1 (16-oz.) pkg. frozen blackberries

1 (16-oz.) pkg. frozen blueberries

1 (10-in.) store-bought angel food cake

1. In a large skillet over medium-high heat, combine sugar, cornstarch, cinnamon, apple juice, and water, whisking to avoid clumps.
2. Add blackberries and blueberries, and bring to a boil. Cook for about 5 minutes or until thickened.
3. Cut angel food cake into 1-inch slices, top with ½ cup berry mixture, and enjoy warm.

Variation: You could also refrigerate the berry mixture to enjoy later over reduced-fat frozen yogurt.

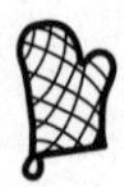

COOLER TALK

It is not well documented where the name "angel food cake" originated, but it is speculated that the cake was unintentionally developed from leftover egg whites after noodle-making.

Fruit Bake

This fruit bake is soft on the inside and crunchy all around with a nice flavor, thanks to the brown sugar and cinnamon.

Yield:	**Prep time:**	**Cook time:**	**Serving size:**
6 cups	15 minutes	25 minutes	$^3/_4$ cup
Each serving has:			
80 calories	17 g carbohydrates	1 g fat	2 g fiber
1 g protein			

2 large apples (your favorite), cored and diced

2 medium peaches, skin on, pitted, and diced

2 TB. slivered almonds

1 cup quick-cooking oats

2 TB. honey

$^1/_2$ tsp. ground cinnamon

1 tsp. vanilla extract

1. Preheat the oven to 375°F. Line a baking sheet with parchment paper.
2. In a large bowl, combine apples, peaches, almonds, quick-cooking oats, honey, cinnamon, and vanilla extract. Transfer to the prepared baking sheet, and spread into an even layer.
3. Bake for 25 minutes. Serve warm with 1 scoop low-fat frozen yogurt on top or cold as a topping for oatmeal or fat-free yogurt.

ACID ALERT

Peaches may trigger reflux in some people. If your food journals indicate that peaches are a problem food for you, substitute bananas instead, or double the amount of apples.

Simple Baked Apples with Frozen Yogurt

The frozen yogurt starts melting as soon as it hits the warm and flavorful baked apples. Brown sugar, cinnamon, vanilla—enough said.

Yield: 2 apples	**Prep time:** 10 minutes	**Cook time:** 10 minutes	**Serving size:** 1 apple
Each serving has:			
264 calories	60 g carbohydrates	2 g fat	5 g fiber
5 g protein			

2 medium apples (your favorite)
1 TB. honey
1 tsp. vanilla extract
¼ tsp. ground cinnamon
⅛ tsp. ground ginger
1 cup low-fat vanilla frozen yogurt

1. Using an apple corer or a small paring knife, core apples, leaving the bottom intact.
2. Spread honey, vanilla extract, cinnamon, and ginger inside apples.
3. Place apples in a microwave-safe dish, and cook on high for 10 minutes or until apples are soft when pierced with a fork.
4. Fill each apple with ½ cup vanilla frozen yogurt, and serve.

Variation: Consider using Banana Ice Cream (recipe later in this chapter) instead of the vanilla frozen yogurt in this recipe.

ACID ALERT

Unless you've been instructed otherwise by your physician, steer clear of sugar-free products and highly processed ice creams. They frequently contain sugar alcohols and other additives that may produce gas, diarrhea, and intestinal discomfort.

Fruit Kebobs

This dessert is warm and slightly browned on the outside and juicy and sweet on the inside. It's a perfect summertime treat.

Yield:	Prep time:	Cook time:	Serving size:
8 kebabs	20 minutes	10 minutes	2 kebabs
Each serving has:			
122 calories	31 g carbohydrates	0 g fat	3 g fiber
2 g protein			

1½ cups honeydew melon

1½ cups cubed cantaloupe

2 medium bananas, peeled and cut into ½-in. medallions

2 TB. dark brown sugar

¼ tsp. ground cinnamon

1. Preheat the broiler to high or heat a grill to high. Soak 8 wooden skewers in water for at least 10 minutes to prevent them from burning in the oven or on the grill.
2. In a medium bowl, combine honeydew melon, cantaloupe, and bananas. Add dark brown sugar and cinnamon, and toss to coat.
3. Distribute fruit equally among 8 skewers.
4. Wrap open ends of the skewers in aluminum foil to prevent burning, and place skewers under the broiler or on the grill. Cook for 3 or 4 minutes per side, rotating frequently to ensure even browning. Enjoy warm.

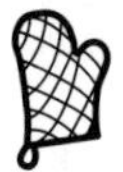

COOLER TALK

Fruit starts turning brown seconds after being exposed to air due to oxidation. You can prevent this process by sprinkling fruit with lemon juice or submerging it in water. The browned fruit, however, is perfectly safe to eat.

Fruit Salad with Coconut

This fresh and juicy salad is perfect for any time of year. The tropical flavor will take your taste buds to an instant vacation getaway.

Yield:	**Prep time:**	**Chill time:**	**Serving size:**
4 cups	10 minutes	1 hour or overnight	1 cup
Each serving has:			
124 calories	30 g carbohydrates	1 g fat	3 g fiber
1 g protein			

1½ cups cubed bananas

1½ cups cubed and peeled papaya

1 cup cubed cantaloupe

2 TB. finely chopped dried apples

2 TB. shredded unsweetened coconut

1 TB. honey

1. In a large bowl, combine bananas, papaya, cantaloupe, dried apples, unsweetened coconut, and honey.
2. Refrigerate for at least 1 hour or overnight. Serve chilled in a large bowl.

TUMMY TAMER

A large cantaloupe has only 300 calories. It's also loaded with vitamins A and C and potassium and is high in vitamin B_6. If hunger strikes, slice a melon in half, scoop out the seeds, and eat with a spoon. Easy and delicious.

Banana Ice Cream

It's hard to believe you can make this creamy and sweet treat at home from just two ingredients!

Yield:	**Prep time:**	**Freeze time:**	**Serving size:**
2 cups	5 minutes	4 hours	1 cup
Each serving has:			
112 calories	28 g carbohydrates	0 g fat	3 g fiber
2 g protein			

2 bananas, peeled and roughly chopped

3 TB. fat-free milk

1. Place chopped bananas in individual zipper-lock bags, and freeze for at least 4 hours or longer.
2. In a blender, combine bananas and fat-free milk. Blend for 2 minutes or until smooth. Serve chilled in small serving bowls.

Variation: If you like a little spice in your life, add $\frac{1}{8}$ teaspoon ground ginger during the blending step.

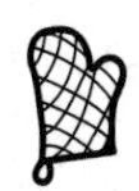

COOLER TALK

Bananas are a great source of potassium and can be used as a snack, added to your oatmeal, or used in many baked goods.

Cherry Almond Balls

Sweet and chewy, these cherry and puffed rice treats are perfect all year round.

Yield:	**Prep time:**	**Cook time:**	**Serving size:**
16 balls	20 minutes, plus 1 or 2 hours chill time	15 minutes	1 ball
Each serving has:			
123 calories	27 g carbohydrates	2 g fat	1 g fiber
2 g protein			

1 (10-oz.) pkg. mini marshmallows

1 TB. light butter

4 cups puffed cereal

$\frac{1}{2}$ cup slivered almonds

1 tsp. vanilla extract

1 cup dried cherries

1. In a medium saucepan over medium-high heat, combine mini marshmallows and light butter, and stir until melted.
2. Fold in puffed cereal, almonds, vanilla extract, and dried cherries. Remove from heat.
3. Line a cookie sheet with parchment paper, and spread cherry mixture on the cookie sheet in a thin layer. Refrigerate for 1 or 2 hours or overnight.
4. Remove the cookie sheet from the refrigerator, and mold mixture into 16 (1-inch) balls. Enjoy immediately or store in the refrigerator for later.

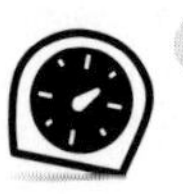

TUMMY TAMER

This is a fun and easy recipe to prepare with kids. It's slightly messy, but the little ones will probably think that makes the process even more enjoyable.

Coconut Date Logs

Sweet and *exotic* are two of the best words to describe these coconut and date treats.

Yield: 8 logs	**Prep time:** 10 minutes	**Serving size:** 1 log
Each serving has:		
38 calories	8 g carbohydrates	1 g fat
1 g fiber	0 g protein	

10 pitted dates

4 TB. unsweetened shredded coconut

1. Place dates and shredded coconut in a small container, and using a handheld blender, purée for 5 minutes or until smooth. (Alternatively, place them in a food processor and purée until smooth.)
2. Form mixture into 8 rectangular logs approximately 1 inch long and $\frac{1}{2}$ inch in diameter. Place on a plate and enjoy.

Variation: For something a little fancier, consider pressing 1 raw almond into the center of each log.

TUMMY TAMER

Dates are a great source of tannins, a substance that's been shown to have anti-inflammatory properties.

Yummy Oatmeal Raisin Cookies

These chewy cookies are filled with oatmeal and raisins to satisfy a sweet-tooth craving.

Yield:	**Prep time:**	**Cook time:**	**Serving size:**
20 cookies	15 minutes	12 minutes	1 cookie
Each serving has:			
130 calories	29 g carbohydrates	1 g fat	2 g fiber
3 g protein			

½ cup whole-wheat pastry flour
½ cup all-purpose flour
1 tsp. baking powder
¼ tsp. ground cinnamon
½ tsp. baking soda
1 cup brown sugar, firmly packed
¼ cup apple butter
2 large egg whites
1 tsp. vanilla extract
2½ cups old-fashioned oats
1 cup raisins

1. Preheat the oven to 350°F. Spray a cookie sheet with nonstick cooking spray.
2. In a medium bowl, combine whole-wheat pastry flour, all-purpose flour, baking powder, cinnamon, baking soda, brown sugar, apple butter, egg whites, vanilla extract, and old-fashioned oats. Using an electric mixer on medium speed, blend for about 1 or 2 minutes or until well mixed.
3. Add raisins, and mix well.
4. Form mixture into 20 (1-inch) balls, and place on the prepared cookie sheet. Bake for 12 minutes per batch.

TUMMY TAMER

Be sure not to overbake these cookies so they maintain their chewiness and moistness on the inside.

Pistachio Meringues

The sweetness of these meringues beautifully complements the saltiness and the crunchiness of the pistachio nuts.

Yield:	Prep time:	Cook time:	Serving size:
36 meringues	15 minutes	1¾ hours	2 meringues
Each serving has:			
73 calories	10 g carbohydrates	3 g fat	1 g fiber
2 g protein			

2 large egg whites

¼ tsp. cream of tartar

¾ cup sugar

1 cup shelled whole pistachio nuts

1. Preheat the oven to 200°F. Line a cookie sheet with parchment paper.
2. In a large bowl, and using an electric mixer on medium speed, beat egg whites and cream of tartar for about 5 minutes or until soft peaks begin to form.
3. Add sugar, and continue beating until stiff peaks form.
4. Fold in pistachio nuts, and mix well.
5. Drop cookies, 1 tablespoon at a time, onto the prepared cookie sheet. Bake for 1¾ hours. Allow cookies to cool completely before serving.

TUMMY TAMER

Pistachio nuts are an excellent source of vitamin E, B-complex vitamins, copper, manganese, potassium, calcium, iron, magnesium, zinc, and selenium. You could eat about 22 to 24 pistachios before reaching 100 calories.

Crepes with Sautéed Apples

These thin and golden crepes pair amazingly well with slightly sweet sautéed apples.

Yield:	**Prep time:**	**Cook time:**	**Serving size:**
8 crepes	10 minutes	20 minutes	2 crepes
Each serving has:			
170 calories	28 g carbohydrates	4 g fat	3 g fiber
5 g protein			

- 3 TB. light butter
- 3 large eggs
- 1 cup fat-free milk
- ¼ tsp. salt
- 1 cup sifted all-purpose flour
- 4 large apples (your favorite), skin on, cored, and sliced thin
- 2 TB. brown sugar
- ¼ tsp. ground cinnamon
- ⅛ tsp. ground ginger
- 1 tsp. confectioners' sugar (optional)

1. In a 9-inch nonstick skillet over medium heat, melt 1 tablespoon light butter.
2. In a medium bowl, whisk together eggs, fat-free milk, salt, and all-purpose flour.
3. Pour ¼ cup batter into the skillet, and rotate the skillet to evenly spread batter. Cook for about 30 seconds. When bubbles start to form on one side, use a spatula to flip over crepe and cook the opposite side for 30 more seconds. Repeat with remaining batter.
4. When crepes are done, increase heat to high, and add remaining 2 tablespoons butter to the skillet. Add apples, brown sugar, cinnamon, and ginger, and cook, stirring frequently, for about 5 minutes or until golden brown.
5. Spread apple mixture evenly among 8 crepes, and serve 2 crepes per plate. Sprinkle with confectioners' sugar (if using), and serve warm.

ACID ALERT

Crepes are often served with many acid reflux trigger foods such as chocolate hazelnut spreads and acidic fruits. Instead, make your own flavor fillings or simply sprinkle with confectioners' sugar for a sweet and safe topping.

Beanie-Greenie Brownies

These yummy brownies hide many healthy ingredients, including beans, but they're so delicious, your taste buds won't even notice.

Yield:	**Prep time:**	**Cook time:**	**Serving size:**
48 brownies	10 minutes	40 minutes	1 brownie
Each serving has:			
110 calories	20 g carbohydrates	4 g fat	2 g fiber
2 g protein			

5 TB. Earth Balance buttery spread

1½ cups unsweetened carob chips

¼ cup tahini

1 cup whipped avocado (easily done with a blender or an immersion blender)

¾ cup puréed cooked beans (your favorite)

1 tsp. baking powder

1 tsp. baking soda

1 cup whole-wheat pastry flour

¼ cup oat flour

1 cup carob powder

2 cups agave syrup

1 TB. vanilla extract

1 cup chopped walnuts

1. Preheat the oven to 325°F. Generously grease a 9×13-inch pan with 2 tablespoons Earth Balance buttery spread.
2. In a large bowl, combine carob chips, remaining 3 tablespoons Earth Balance spread, and tahini.
3. Fill a medium saucepan half full of water, and bring to a boil over high heat. Turn off heat, and set the bowl with carob mixture over hot water. Whisk melting carob mixture until smooth.
4. Remove the bowl from the pan, and whisk in whipped avocado and puréed beans until incorporated.
5. In a medium bowl, combine baking powder, baking soda, whole-wheat pastry flour, oat flour, and carob powder.
6. In a small bowl, combine agave syrup and vanilla extract.

7. Using an electric mixer on medium speed, combine ingredients by alternating adding $^1/_2$ cup at a time of dry ingredients and agave mixture to batter.

8. Fold in walnuts, and spread batter into the prepared pan. Bake for 40 minutes or until a cake tester inserted into the center reveals moist crumbs. Cool for 40 minutes before cutting and serving.

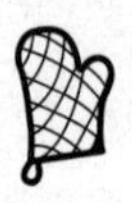

COOLER TALK

This recipe was published in *101 Optimal Life Foods* by David Grotto, RD, LDN. The original recipe was created by Deb Schiff, author of the blog Altered Plates (alteredplates.blogspot.com).

Glossary

Appendix

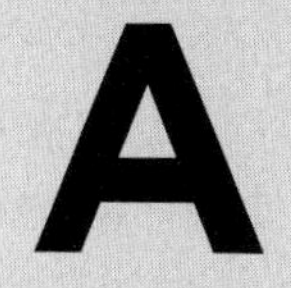

agar agar A gelling agent traditionally used in Asian cuisine for making desserts. Agar is derived from red algae. Its gelling capability and bland flavor make it a versatile ingredient in not only desserts but also soups, sauces, and gravies.

al dente Italian for "against the teeth." Refers to pasta or rice that's neither soft nor hard, but just slightly firm against the teeth.

all-purpose flour Flour that contains only the inner part of the wheat grain. Usable for all purposes, from cakes to gravies.

allspice Named for its flavor echoes of several spices (cinnamon, cloves, nutmeg), allspice is used in many desserts and in rich marinades and stews.

almonds Mild, sweet, and crunchy nuts that combine nicely with creamy and sweet food items.

anchovies (also **sardines**) Tiny, flavorful, preserved fish that typically come in cans. Anchovies are a traditional garnish for Caesar salad, the dressing of which contains anchovy paste.

arborio rice A plump Italian rice used, among other purposes, for risotto.

artichoke hearts The center part of the artichoke flower, often found canned in grocery stores.

arugula A spicy-peppery garden plant with leaves that resemble a dandelion and have a distinctive—and very sharp—flavor.

au gratin The quick broiling of a dish before serving to brown the top ingredients. When used in a recipe name, the term often implies cheese and a creamy sauce.

bake To cook in a dry oven. Dry-heat cooking often results in a crisping of the exterior of the food being cooked. Moist-heat cooking, through methods such as steaming, poaching, etc., brings a much different, moist quality to the food.

baking powder A dry ingredient used to increase volume and lighten or leaven baked goods.

balsamic vinegar Vinegar produced primarily in Italy from a specific type of grape and aged in wood barrels. It is heavier, darker, and sweeter than most vinegars.

bamboo shoots The crunchy, tasty white parts of the growing bamboo plant, often purchased canned.

barbecue To quick-cook over high heat, or to cook something long and slow in a rich liquid (barbecue sauce).

basil A flavorful, almost sweet, resinous herb delicious with tomatoes and used in all kinds of Italian or Mediterranean-style dishes.

baste To keep foods moist during cooking by spooning, brushing, or drizzling with a liquid.

beat To quickly mix substances.

blackening To cook something quickly in a very hot skillet over high heat, usually with a seasoning mixture. Cajun cooking makes frequent use of blackening.

blanch To place a food in boiling water for about 1 minute (or less) to partially cook the exterior and then submerge in or rinse with cool water to halt the cooking.

blend To completely mix something, usually with a blender or food processor, more slowly than beating.

blue cheese A blue-veined cheese that crumbles easily and has a somewhat soft texture, usually sold in a block. The color is from a flavorful, edible mold that is often added or injected into the cheese.

boil To heat a liquid to the point where water is forced to turn into steam, causing the liquid to bubble. To boil something is to insert it into boiling water. A rapid boil is when a lot of bubbles form on the surface of the liquid.

bok choy (also **Chinese cabbage**) A member of the cabbage family with thick stems, crisp texture, and fresh flavor. It's perfect for stir-frying.

bouillon Dried essence of stock from chicken, beef, vegetables, or other ingredients. This is a popular starting ingredient for soups as it adds flavor (and often a lot of salt).

braise To cook with the introduction of some liquid, usually over an extended period of time.

breadcrumbs Tiny pieces of crumbled dry bread, often used for topping or coating.

Brie A creamy cow's milk cheese from France with a soft, edible rind and a mild flavor.

brine A highly salted, often seasoned, liquid used to flavor and preserve foods. To brine a food is to soak, or preserve, it by submerging it in brine. The salt in the brine penetrates the fibers of meat and makes it moist and tender.

broil To cook in a dry oven under the overhead high-heat element.

broth *See* stock.

brown To cook in a skillet, turning, until the food's surface is seared and brown in color, to lock in the juices.

brown rice Whole-grain rice including the germ with a characteristic pale brown or tan color; more nutritious and flavorful than white rice.

bruschetta (or **crostini**) Slices of toasted or grilled bread with garlic and olive oil, often with other toppings.

bulgur A wheat kernel that's been steamed, dried, and crushed and is sold in fine and coarse textures.

cake flour Flour that's lower in protein content than all-purpose flour. It's commonly used for making cakes and pastry, hence the name, because it produces a tenderer product.

capers Flavorful buds of a Mediterranean plant, ranging in size from *nonpareil* (about the size of a small pea) to larger, grape-size caper berries produced in Spain.

caramelize To cook sugar over low heat until it develops a sweet caramel flavor. The term is increasingly used to describe cooking vegetables (especially onions) or meat in butter or oil over low heat until they soften, sweeten, and develop a caramel color.

caraway A distinctive spicy seed used for bread, pork, cheese, and cabbage dishes. It is known to reduce stomach upset, which is why it is often paired with, for example, sauerkraut.

carbohydrate A nutritional component found in starches, sugars, fruits, and vegetables that causes a rise in blood glucose levels. Carbohydrates supply energy and many important nutrients, including vitamins, minerals, and antioxidants.

cardamom An intense, sweet-smelling spice used in baking and coffee and common in Indian cooking.

cayenne A fiery spice made from (hot) chili peppers, especially the cayenne chili, a slender, red, and very hot pepper.

ceviche A seafood dish in which fresh fish or seafood is marinated for several hours in highly acidic lemon or lime juice, tomato, onion, and cilantro. The acid "cooks" the seafood.

cheddar The ubiquitous hard cow's milk cheese with a rich, buttery flavor that ranges from mellow to sharp. Originally produced in England, cheddar is now produced worldwide.

chevre French for "goat cheese," chevre is a typically creamy-salty soft cheese delicious by itself or paired with fruits or chutney. Chevres vary in style from mild and creamy to aged, firm, and flavorful.

chickpeas (or garbanzo beans) Yellow-gold, roundish beans used as the base ingredient in hummus. Chickpeas are high in fiber and low in fat.

chili powder A seasoning blend that includes chili pepper, cumin, garlic, and oregano. Proportions vary among different versions, but they all offer a warm, rich flavor.

chilis (or **chiles**) Any one of many different "hot" peppers, ranging in intensity from the relatively mild ancho pepper to the blisteringly hot habañero.

Chinese five-spice powder A seasoning blend of cinnamon, anise, ginger, fennel, and pepper.

chives A member of the onion family, chives grow in bunches of long leaves that resemble tall grass or the green tops of onions and offer a light onion flavor.

chop To cut into pieces, usually qualified by an adverb such as "*coarsely* chopped" or by a size measurement such as "chopped into $^1/_2$-inch pieces." "Finely chopped" is much closer to mince.

chutney A thick condiment often served with Indian curries made with fruits and/or vegetables with vinegar, sugar, and spices.

chyme A semifluid consisting of partially digested food, gastric juices, and digestive enzymes. Chyme passes from the stomach into the small intestine for further digestion.

cider vinegar Vinegar produced from apple cider, popular in North America.

cilantro A member of the parsley family used in Mexican cooking (especially salsa) and some Asian dishes. Use in moderation, as the flavor can overwhelm. The seed of the cilantro is the spice coriander.

cinnamon A rich, aromatic spice commonly used in baking or desserts. Cinnamon can also be used for delicious and interesting entrées.

clove A sweet, strong, almost wintergreen-flavor spice used in baking and with meats such as ham.

compote A chilled dish of fresh or dried fruit that's slowly cooked in a sugary syrup made of liquid and spices.

coriander A rich, warm, spicy seed used in all types of recipes, from African to South American, from entrées to desserts.

cornstarch A thickener used in baking and food processing. It's the refined starch of the endosperm of the corn kernel and often mixed with cold liquid to make into a paste before adding to a recipe to avoid clumps.

count In terms of seafood or other foods that come in small sizes, the number of that item that compose 1 pound. For example, 31- to 40-count shrimp are large appetizer shrimp often served with cocktail sauce; 51 to 60 are much smaller.

couscous Granular semolina (durum wheat) that is cooked and used in many Mediterranean and North African dishes.

cream To beat a fat such as butter, often with another ingredient such as sugar, to soften and aerate a batter.

crimini mushrooms A relative of the white button mushroom that is brown in color and has a richer flavor. The larger, fully grown version is the portobello. *See also* portobello mushrooms.

croutons Chunks of bread, usually between $\frac{1}{4}$ and $\frac{1}{2}$ inch in size, sometimes seasoned and baked, broiled, or fried to a crisp texture and used in soups and salads.

cumin A fiery, smoky-tasting spice popular in Middle Eastern and Indian dishes. Cumin is a seed; ground cumin seed is the most common form used in cooking.

curd A gelatinous substance resulting from coagulated milk used to make cheese. Curd also refers to dishes of similar texture, such as dishes made with egg (lemon curd).

curry Rich, spicy, Indian-style sauces and the dishes prepared with them. A curry uses curry powder as its base seasoning.

curry powder A ground blend of rich and flavorful spices used as a basis for curry and many other Indian-influenced dishes. Common ingredients include hot pepper, nutmeg, cumin, cinnamon, pepper, and turmeric. Some curry can also be found in paste form.

custard A cooked mixture of eggs and milk popular as a base for desserts.

dash A few drops, usually of a liquid, released by a quick shake of, for example, a bottle of hot sauce.

deglaze To scrape up the bits of meat and seasoning left in a pan or skillet after cooking. Usually this is done by adding a liquid such as wine or broth and creating a flavorful stock that can be used to create sauces.

dice To cut into small cubes about $\frac{1}{4}$-inch square.

Dijon mustard Hearty, spicy mustard made in the style of the Dijon region of France.

dill A herb perfect for eggs, salmon, cheese dishes, and, of course, vegetables (pickles!).

dollop A spoonful of something creamy and thick, like sour cream or whipped cream.

double boiler A set of two pots designed to nest together, one inside the other, and provide consistent, moist heat for foods that need delicate treatment. The bottom pot holds water (not quite touching the bottom of the top pot); the top pot holds the food you want to heat.

dredge To cover a piece of food with a dry substance such as flour or corn meal.

drizzle To lightly sprinkle drops of a liquid over food, often as the finishing touch to a dish.

edamame Fresh, plump, pale green soybeans, similar in appearance to lima beans, often served steamed and either shelled or still in their protective pods.

electrolytes Substances that give the body the capacity to conduct electricity, an essential function for our cells and organs. A typical electrolyte solution contains sodium, potassium, and chloride.

emulsion A combination of liquid ingredients that do not normally mix well beaten together to create a thick liquid, such as a fat or oil with water. Creation of an emulsion must be done carefully and rapidly to ensure that particles of one ingredient are suspended in the other.

en papillote A cooking method wherein the food is placed in a folded pouch, normally parchment-type paper. The pouch is tightly sealed to create a closed environment that will help steam the food while preserving the flavor.

endive A green that resembles a small, elongated, tightly packed head of romaine lettuce. The thick, crunchy leaves can be broken off and used with dips and spreads.

entrée The main dish in a meal. In France, however, the entrée is considered the first course.

extra-virgin olive oil *See* olive oil.

extract A concentrated flavoring derived from foods or plants through evaporation or distillation that imparts a powerful flavor without altering the volume or texture of a dish.

falafel A Middle Eastern food made of seasoned, ground chickpeas formed into balls, cooked, and often used as a filling in pitas.

fennel In seed form, a fragrant, licorice-tasting herb. The bulbs have a much milder flavor and a celery-like crunch and are used as a vegetable in salads or cooked recipes.

feta A white, crumbly, sharp, and salty cheese popular in Greek cooking and on salads. Traditional feta is usually made with sheep's milk, but feta-style cheese can be made from sheep's, cow's, or goat's milk.

fillet A piece of meat or seafood with the bones removed.

flake To break into thin sections, as with fish.

floret The flower or bud end of broccoli or cauliflower.

flour Grains ground into a meal. Wheat is perhaps the most common flour. Flour is also made from oats, rye, buckwheat, soybeans, etc. *See also* all-purpose flour; cake flour; whole-wheat flour.

fold To combine a dense and light mixture with a circular action from the middle of the bowl.

food diary A record of what foods you've eaten, how much, and at what time. Keeping a food diary can be helpful in identifying acid reflux triggers.

fricassee A dish, usually chicken, cut into pieces and cooked in a liquid or sauce.

frittata A skillet-cooked mixture of eggs and other ingredients that's not stirred but is cooked slowly and then either flipped or finished under the broiler.

fry *See* sauté.

garlic A member of the onion family, a pungent and flavorful element in many savory dishes. A garlic bulb contains multiple cloves. Each clove, when chopped, provides about 1 teaspoon garlic. Most recipes call for cloves or chopped garlic by the teaspoon.

garnish An embellishment not vital to the dish but added to enhance visual appeal.

gastric motility The movement of the stomach that helps direct contents from the stomach to the small intestines.

gazpacho A cold, uncooked soup originating in Spain that's a puréed mixture of tomatoes, bell peppers, onions, celery, and cucumber.

ginger Available in fresh root or dried, ground form, ginger adds a pungent, sweet, and spicy quality to a dish.

Gorgonzola A creamy and rich Italian blue cheese. "Dolce" is sweet, and that's the kind you want.

grate To shave into tiny pieces using a sharp rasp or grater.

Greek yogurt A strained yogurt that's a good natural source of protein, calcium, and probiotics. On average, Greek yogurt contains 40 percent more protein per ounce than traditional yogurt.

grind To reduce a large, hard substance, often a seasoning such as peppercorns, to the consistency of sand.

Gruyère A rich, sharp cow's milk cheese made in Switzerland that has a nutty flavor.

handful An unscientific measurement, the amount of an ingredient you can hold in your hand.

Havarti A creamy, Danish, mild cow's milk cheese perhaps most enjoyed in its herbed versions such as Havarti with dill.

hazelnuts (also **filberts**) A sweet nut popular in desserts and, to a lesser degree, in savory dishes.

hearts of palm Firm, elongated, off-white cylinders from the inside of a palm tree stem tip.

herbes de Provence A seasoning mix including basil, fennel, marjoram, rosemary, sage, and thyme, common in the south of France.

hoisin sauce A sweet Asian condiment similar to ketchup made with soybeans, sesame, chili peppers, and sugar.

horseradish A sharp, spicy root that forms the flavor base in many condiments from cocktail sauce to sharp mustards. Prepared horseradish contains vinegar and oil, among other ingredients. Use pure horseradish much more sparingly than the prepared version, or try cutting it with sour cream.

hummus A thick, Middle Eastern spread made of puréed chickpeas, lemon juice, olive oil, garlic, and often tahini (sesame seed paste).

hyperosmolarity The increased osmotic concentration of a solution.

hypoglycemia A condition in which a person has an abnormally low level of blood sugar. It can result from prolonged exercise, poor diet, or excessive insulin production.

infusion A liquid in which flavorful ingredients such as herbs have been soaked or steeped to extract that flavor into the liquid.

Italian seasoning A blend of dried herbs, including basil, oregano, rosemary, and thyme.

jicama A juicy, crunchy, sweet, large, round Central American vegetable. If you can't find jicama, try substituting sliced water chestnuts.

julienne A French word meaning "to slice into very thin pieces."

kalamata olives Traditionally from Greece, these medium-small, long black olives have a smoky rich flavor.

Key limes Very small limes grown primarily in Florida known for their tart taste.

knead To work dough to make it pliable so it holds gas bubbles as it bakes. Kneading is fundamental in the process of making yeast breads.

kosher salt A coarse-grained salt made without any additives or iodine.

lentils Tiny lens-shape pulses used in European, Middle Eastern, and Indian cuisines.

macerate To mix sugar or another sweetener with fruit. The fruit softens, and its juice is released to mix with the sweetener.

marinate To soak meat, seafood, or another food in a seasoned sauce, called a marinade, which is high in acid content. The acids break down the muscle of a meat, making it tender and adding flavor.

marjoram A sweet herb, cousin of and similar to oregano, popular in Greek, Spanish, and Italian dishes.

mascarpone A thick, creamy, spreadable cheese, traditionally from Italy.

meld To allow flavors to blend and spread over time. Melding is often why recipes call for overnight refrigeration and is also why some dishes taste better as leftovers.

meringue A baked mixture of sugar and beaten egg whites, often used as a dessert topping. Sometimes, some cookies are called meringues.

mesclun Mixed salad greens, usually containing lettuce and assorted greens such as arugula, cress, endive, and others.

millet A tiny, round, yellow-colored nutty-flavored grain often used as a replacement for couscous.

mince To cut into very small pieces smaller than diced pieces, about $\frac{1}{8}$ inch or smaller.

miso A fermented, flavorful soybean paste, key in many Japanese dishes.

mouthfeel The overall sensation in the mouth resulting from a combination of the temperature, taste, smell, and texture of the food.

nutmeg A sweet, fragrant, musky spice used primarily in baking.

olive oil A fragrant liquid produced by crushing or pressing olives. Extra-virgin olive oil—the most flavorful and highest quality—is produced from the first pressing of a batch of olives; oil is also produced from later pressings.

olives The fruit of the olive tree commonly grown on all sides of the Mediterranean. Black olives are also called ripe olives. Green olives are immature, although they are also widely eaten. *See also* kalamata olives.

omelet A breakfast dish made of beaten eggs that are cooked until set. It's often folded and has a filling such as meat, vegetables, or cheese.

oregano A fragrant, slightly astringent herb used in Greek, Spanish, and Italian dishes.

orzo A rice-shape pasta used in Greek cooking.

oxidation The browning of fruit flesh that happens over time and with exposure to air. Minimize oxidation by rubbing the cut surfaces with a lemon half. Oxidation also affects wine, which is why the taste changes over time after a bottle is opened.

paella A grand Spanish dish of rice, shellfish, onion, meats, rich broth, and herbs.

paprika A rich, red, warm, earthy spice that also lends a rich red color to many dishes.

parboil To partially cook in boiling water or broth, similar to blanching (although blanched foods are quickly cooled with cold water).

Parmesan A hard, dry, flavorful cheese primarily used grated or shredded as a seasoning for Italian-style dishes.

parsley A fresh-tasting green leafy herb, often used as a garnish.

pâté A savory loaf that contains meats, poultry, or seafood; spices; and often a lot of fat. It's served cold and spread or sliced on crusty bread or crackers.

pecans Rich, buttery nuts, native to North America, that have a high unsaturated fat content.

peppercorns Large, round, dried berries ground to produce pepper.

peristalsis A medical term that describes the smooth, rhythmic, wavelike contractions of the intestines that propel contents through the digestive tract.

pesto A thick spread or sauce made with fresh basil leaves, garlic, olive oil, pine nuts, and Parmesan cheese. Some newer versions are made with other herbs.

pickle A food, usually a vegetable such as a cucumber, that's been pickled in brine.

pilaf A rice dish in which the rice is browned in butter or oil and then cooked in a flavorful liquid such as a broth, often with the addition of meats or vegetables. The rice absorbs the broth, resulting in a savory dish.

pinch An unscientific measurement, the amount of an ingredient—typically a dry, granular substance such as an herb or seasoning—you can hold between your finger and thumb.

pine nuts (also **pignoli** or **piñon**) Nuts grown on pine trees that are rich (read: high in fat), flavorful, and a bit pine-y. Pine nuts are a traditional component of pesto and add a wonderful hearty crunch to many other recipes.

pita bread A flat, hollow wheat bread often used for sandwiches or sliced, pizza style. They're terrific soft with dips or baked or broiled as a vehicle for other ingredients.

pizza stone Preheated with the oven, a pizza stone cooks a crust to a delicious, crispy, pizza-parlor texture. It also holds heat well, so a pizza or other food removed from the oven on the stone stays hot for as long as a half hour at the table. Great for cooking method that uses minimal to no oil, ideal for acid reflux sufferers.

plyometrics A type of physical training style designed to produce explosive, rapid, and powerful movements for the purpose of improving sports performance. It is not advised for acid reflux sufferers.

poach To cook a food in simmering liquid such as water, wine, or broth.

polenta A mush made from cornmeal that can be eaten hot with butter or cooked until firm and cut into squares.

porcini mushrooms Rich and flavorful mushrooms used in rice and Italian-style dishes.

portobello mushrooms A mature and larger form of the smaller crimini mushroom, portobellos are brownish, chewy, and flavorful. Often served as whole caps, grilled, or as thin sautéed slices. *See also* crimini mushrooms.

preheat To turn on an oven, broiler, or other cooking appliance in advance of cooking so the temperature will be at the desired level when the assembled dish is ready for cooking.

proof To place yeast in warm water and allow it to start producing bubbly foam. This indicates the yeast is active.

prosciutto Dry, salt-cured ham that originated in Italy.

purée To reduce a food to a thick, creamy texture, typically using a blender or food processor.

quinoa A nutty-flavored grain that's extremely high in protein and calcium.

reduce To boil or simmer a broth or sauce to remove some of the water content, resulting in more concentrated flavor and color.

render To cook a meat to the point where its fat melts and can be removed.

reserve To hold a specified ingredient for another use later in the recipe.

rice vinegar Vinegar produced from fermented rice or rice wine, popular in Asian-style dishes. Different from rice wine vinegar.

ricotta A fresh Italian cheese that's smoother than cottage cheese with a slightly sweet flavor.

risotto A popular Italian rice dish made by browning arborio rice in butter or oil and then slowly adding liquid to cook the rice, resulting in a creamy texture.

roast To cook something uncovered in an oven, usually without additional liquid.

Roquefort A world-famous, French, creamy but sharp sheep's milk cheese containing blue lines of mold.

rosemary A pungent, sweet herb used with chicken, pork, fish, and especially lamb. A little of it goes a long way.

roux A mixture of butter or another fat and flour, used to thicken sauces and soups.

rutabaga A vegetable, often confused for turnips, that's a close relative of turnips but technically a mix of turnips and cabbage.

sabazi A word that collectively describes any vegetable dish in Indian cuisine.

saffron A spice made from the stamens of crocus flowers, saffron lends a dramatic yellow color and distinctive flavor to a dish. Use only tiny amounts of this expensive herb.

sage An herb with a musty yet fruity, lemon-rind scent and "sunny" flavor.

salsa A style of mixing fresh vegetables and/or fresh fruit in a coarse chop. Salsa can be spicy or not, fruit-based or not, and served as a starter on its own (with chips, for example) or as a companion to a main course.

sauté To pan-cook over lower heat than used for frying.

savory A popular herb with a fresh, woody taste. Can also describe the flavor of food, resembling the taste of savory.

scald To heat milk just until it's about to boil and then remove it from heat. Scalding milk helps prevent it from souring.

scant An ingredient measurement directive not to add any extra, perhaps even leaving the measurement a tad short.

Scoville scale A scale used to measure the "hot" in hot peppers. The lower the Scoville units, the more mild the pepper. Mildly hot ancho peppers are about 3,000 Scovilles; Tears of Fire and habañero peppers are 30,000 Scovilles or more.

sear To quickly brown the exterior of a food, especially meat, over high heat to preserve interior moisture.

sesame oil An oil, made from pressing sesame seeds, that's tasteless if clear and aromatic and flavorful if brown.

shallot A member of the onion family that grows in a bulb somewhat like garlic but has a milder onion flavor. When a recipe calls for shallot, use the entire bulb.

shellfish A broad range of seafood, including clams, mussels, oysters, crabs, shrimp, and lobster. Some people are allergic to shellfish, so take care with its inclusion in recipes.

shiitake mushrooms Large, dark brown mushrooms with a hearty, meaty flavor. Can be used either fresh or dried, grilled or as a component in other recipes, and as a flavoring source for broth.

short-grain rice A starchy rice popular for Asian-style dishes because it readily clumps (perfect for eating with chopsticks).

shred To cut into many long, thin slices.

simmer To boil gently so the liquid barely bubbles.

skillet (also **frying pan**) A generally heavy, flat-bottomed, metal pan with a handle designed to cook food over heat on a stovetop or campfire.

skim To remove fat or other material from the top of liquid.

slice To cut into thin pieces.

steam To suspend a food over boiling water and allow the heat of the steam (water vapor) to cook the food. A quick cooking method, steaming preserves the flavor and texture of a food.

steep To let sit in hot water, as in steeping tea in hot water for 10 minutes.

stew To slowly cook pieces of food submerged in a liquid. Also, a dish that has been prepared by this method.

sticky rice (or **glutinous rice**) *See* short-grain rice.

Stilton The famous English blue-veined cheese, delicious with toasted nuts and renowned for its pairing with Port wine.

stir-fry To cook small pieces of food in a wok or skillet over high heat, moving and turning the food quickly to cook all sides.

stock A flavorful broth made by cooking meats and/or vegetables with seasonings until the liquid absorbs these flavors. This liquid is then strained and the solids discarded. Can be eaten alone or used as a base for soups, stews, etc.

strata A savory bread pudding made with eggs and cheese.

succotash A cooked vegetable dish usually made of corn and peppers.

tahini A paste made from sesame seeds used to flavor many Middle Eastern recipes.

tamarind A sweet, pungent, flavorful fruit used in Indian-style sauces and curries.

tapas A Spanish term that collectively describes appetizers and snacks. Tapas can be either cold or warm.

tapenade A thick, chunky spread made from savory ingredients such as olives, lemon juice, and anchovies.

tarragon A sweet, rich-smelling herb perfect with seafood, vegetables (especially asparagus), chicken, and pork.

tempeh An Indonesian food made by culturing and fermenting soybeans into a cake, sometimes mixed with grains or vegetables. It's high in protein and fiber.

teriyaki A Japanese-style sauce composed of soy sauce, rice wine, ginger, and sugar that works well with seafood as well as most meats.

thyme A minty, zesty herb.

toast To heat something, usually bread, so it's browned and crisp.

tofu A cheeselike substance made from soybeans and soy milk.

tomatillo A small, round fruit with a distinctive spicy flavor, often found in south-of-the-border dishes. To use, remove the papery outer skin, rinse off any sticky residue, and chop like a tomato.

turmeric A spicy, pungent, yellow root used in many dishes, especially Indian cuisine, for color and flavor. Turmeric is the source of the yellow color in many prepared mustards.

tzatziki A Greek dip traditionally made with Greek yogurt, cucumbers, garlic, and mint.

veal Meat from a calf, generally characterized by mild flavor and tenderness.

vegetable steamer An insert for a large saucepan or a special pot with tiny holes in the bottom designed to fit on another pot to hold food to be steamed above boiling water. *See also* steam.

vinegar An acidic liquid widely used as a dressing and seasoning, often made from fermented grapes, apples, or rice. *See also* balsamic vinegar; cider vinegar; rice vinegar; white vinegar; wine vinegar.

walnuts A rich, slightly woody flavored nut.

wasabi Japanese horseradish, a fiery, pungent condiment used with many Japanese-style dishes. Most often sold as a powder; add water to create a paste.

water chestnuts A tuber popular in many types of Asian-style cooking. The flesh is white, crunchy, and juicy, and the vegetable holds its texture whether cool or hot.

whisk To rapidly mix, introducing air to the mixture.

white mushrooms Button mushrooms. When fresh, they have an earthy smell and an appealing "soft crunch."

white vinegar The most common type of vinegar, produced from grain.

whole grain A grain derived from the seeds of grasses, including rice, oats, rye, wheat, wild rice, quinoa, barley, buckwheat, bulgur, corn, millet, amaranth, and sorghum.

whole-wheat flour Wheat flour that contains the entire grain.

wild rice Actually a grass with a rich, nutty flavor, it's popular as an unusual and nutritious side dish.

wine vinegar Vinegar produced from red or white wine.

Worcestershire sauce Originally developed in India and containing tamarind, this spicy sauce is used as a seasoning for many meats and other dishes.

yeast Tiny fungi that, when mixed with water, sugar, flour, and heat, release carbon dioxide bubbles, which, in turn, cause the bread to rise.

zest Small slivers of peel, usually from a citrus fruit such as lemon, lime, or orange.

zester A kitchen tool used to scrape zest off a fruit. A small grater also works well.

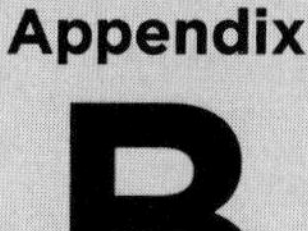

Resources

B

By now, you probably have a good grasp of what acid reflux is and how you can manage your symptoms. But if you need help, or want more information, I've included this list of resources that can help you find the right professional in your area, find reliable information on the web, and discover more books filled with fun recipes to further expand your kitchen repertoire.

Professional Organizations

American Academy of Family Physicians
aafp.org

American College of Gastroenterology
acg.gi.org

American Dietetic Association
eatright.org

American Medical Association
ama-assn.org

American Society for Gastrointestinal Endoscopy
asge.org

FamilyDoctor.org
familydoctor.org

Web Resources

Cleveland Clinic
clevelandclinic.org

Mayo Clinic
mayoclinic.com

National Center for Complementary and Alternative Medicine
nccam.nih.gov

National Digestive Diseases Information Clearinghouse
digestive.niddk.nih.gov

National Restaurant Association Nutrition Resources
restaurant.org/tools/nutrition

Office of Dietary Supplements (National Institutes of Health)
ods.od.nih.gov

RD411
rd411.com

U.S. Pharmacopeia
usp.org

WebMD
webmd.com

Further Reading

King, John. *Mayo Clinic on Digestive Health*. Rochester, MN: Mayo Clinic, 2004.

Sierpina, Victor C. *The Healthy Gut Workbook*. Oakland, CA: New Harbinger Publications, 2010.

Taub-Dix, Bonnie. *Read It Before You Eat It*. New York, NY: Penguin Group USA, 2010.

Wansink, Brian. *Mindless Eating*. New York, NY: Bantam Books, 2010.

Wendland, Barbara. *Chronic Heartburn: Managing Acid Reflux and GERD Through Understanding, Diet and Lifestyle*. Toronto, Ontario, Canada: Robert Rose, 2006.

Index

A

B

C

D

E

F

G

H

I-J-K

L

M

N–O

P

Q–R

T

U-V

W-X

Y–Z